SHAKING MEDICINE

"I had a personal experience of Brad's shaking power. . . . He placed one of his hands on my upper back and the other opposite on my upper chest. He began to shake vigorously, and apparently involuntarily, throughout his entire body. His face, shoulders, torso, and feet were vibrating with some invisible power, like a wave that was continuously cresting in his body and crashing and rippling in his fingertips. I felt the trembling power pass through me. . . . While receiving this beautiful 'gift,' I was transported to the Kalahari. I saw the tribal people with whom he had danced; I viewed their villages and landscape. I was in Africa as truly as if I had opened my eyes and found myself physically there."

KENNETH COHEN, AUTHOR OF *THE WAY OF QIGONG: THE ART AND SCIENCE OF CHINESE ENERGY HEALING*

"Dr. Keeney's work marks the beginning of an awakening of the universal life force that is accessible to everyone. I have personally experienced his method of moving the life force in my own body—circulating it up and down my spine, passing it through my fingertips, and feeling it tingling the tips of my toes. It is time for each of us to become acquainted with this energizing force."

DR. ROBERT FULFORD, AUTHOR OF *DR. FULFORD'S TOUCH OF LIFE: ALIGNING BODY, MIND, AND SPIRIT TO HONOR THE HEALER WITHIN*

"Bradford Keeney is an authentic shaman who, in his ceremonial practice, answers the question: What would happen if you gave a university professor a kind heart and a limitless infusion of spiritual power?"

STEPHEN AND ROBIN LARSEN, AUTHORS OF *A FIRE IN THE MIND: THE LIFE OF JOSEPH CAMPBELL*

"I felt like I was floating and wanted to move my body with speed and precision. All of my senses were intensified. I recognized this condition as being similar to the ki activation that I had learned to utilize in aikido training. The difference was that the intensity of this energy was magnitudes beyond what I had previously experienced; it was beyond what I'd ever imagined."

DON WRIGHT, FORMER TEACHER OF
ERICKSONIAN HYPNOTHERAPY AT THE ESALEN INSTITUTE

"The experience I had in Brad Keeney's ceremony was very important—his hands irradiated light in my head."

DR. PIERRE WEIL, AUTHOR OF
THE ART OF LIVING IN PEACE: TOWARDS
A NEW PEACE CONSCIOUSNESS, FOUNDER OF THE
INTERNATIONAL HOLISTIC UNIVERSITY OF BRASILIA,
AND CONSULTANT TO THE UNITED NATIONS

SHAKING
MEDICINE

THE HEALING POWER OF ECSTATIC MOVEMENT

Bradford Keeney

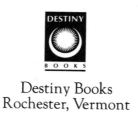

Destiny Books
Rochester, Vermont

Destiny Books
One Park Street
Rochester, Vermont 05767
www.DestinyBooks.com

Destiny Books is a division of Inner Traditions International

Library of Congress Cataloging-in-Publication Data
Keeney, Bradford P.
  Shaking medicine : the healing power of ecstatic movement / Bradford Keeney.
     p. cm.
  Includes bibliographical references and index.
  ISBN-13: 978-1-59477-149-1
  ISBN-10: 1-59477-149-9
  1. Mental healing. 2. Alternative medicine. 3. Healing. 4. Self-care, Health.
I. Title.
  RZ400.K44 2007
  615.8'51—dc22

                                                                    2007004109

Printed and bound in the United States by Lake Book Manufacturing

10 9 8 7 6 5 4 3 2 1

Text design and layout by Jon Desautels
This book was typeset in Sabon with Goudy Old Style as a display typeface

To send correspondence to the author of this book, mail a first-class letter to the author c/o Inner Traditions • Bear & Company, One Park Street, Rochester, VT 05767, and we will forward the communication.

CONTENTS

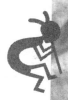

PRONUNCIATION GUIDE

Throughout this book you will notice unusual punctuation marks in words from the Ju|'hoan language of the Kalahari Bushmen. These marks are symbols for the four distinct click sounds used in this language. According to the anthropologist and linguist Megan Biesele, they are pronounced as follows:

| is a dental click that sounds like *tsk, tsk* and is made by putting the tongue behind the teeth.

≠ is an alveolar click, a soft pop made by putting the tongue behind the ridge that is located behind the front teeth.

! is an alveolar-palatal click, a sharp pop made by drawing the tongue down quickly from the roof of the mouth.

‖ is a lateral click, a clucking sound similar to that made by the English when they urge on a horse.

' is a glottal stop, as in the Cockney English pronunciation of *bottle.*

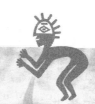

FOREWORD
By the Bushman Elders

We, the elder Bushman shamans of the Kalahari, are descendants of the original custodians of shaking medicine. As members of the ancestral culture for all people on earth, we have always looked after the original forms of healing and communicating with God. All of us are delighted that the words of this book are being brought into the world so that others may know what we have known about shaking medicine since the beginning of human existence.

Over the years, we have been grateful for our relationship with Bradford Keeney, who fully understands and practices our healing and spiritual ways He is a *n|om-kxao,* what we call an owner of *n|om,* the power that makes one shake in deep and meaningful ways. For the Ju|'hoan Bushmen, there are different levels of expertise in the handling of n|om, and we are the last ones entitled to be called *G≠aqba-n!a'an,* the "Heart of the Spears." This title refers to someone who has spent a lifetime growing in n|om and who has received all the healing knowledge and wisdom of God's shaking medicine. We regard Bradford Keeney as a Heart of the Spears.

A Heart of the Spears has been made a master of shaking medicine through experiences and lessons taught by God and the ancestors. We have learned that our minds require the inspiration of a loving heart, and that we should be cautious about the trickster voice of any mind disconnected from the love of God. Medicine, in its highest form, is always poured from God's heart. Please do not consider us the carriers of primitive truths that historically gave way to more evolved ways of thinking, worshipping, and healing. Rather, we hold the purest forms of healing and loving relationships with God, one another, the animals and plants of the world, as well as the earth, water, and sky. In our worldview, First Creation is still present, always ready to breathe its shaking and changing into the stuck world of language, or what we call Second Creation. We, the First People, ask that the world open its heart for a great healing, one that requires the shaking medicine brought about when First Creation and Second Creation interact.

There are many tricksters leading people astray. They almost always use words like "good," "love," "peace," and "God," but make their arguments solely with words printed on paper. For us, the truth a person carries is proved by the way his or her voice and body give way to vibrant sound and song and shaking movements of ecstatic joy. Without seeing, hearing, and feeling a performance of loving medicine, we do not accept anyone's authority to speak about healing wisdom.

We have danced and shaken with Bradford Keeney for many years. He has placed his healing hands on many of us throughout our villages in Namibia and Botswana. We know that he carries truth in his heart, and that his mind, body, and soul shake with the gods and ancestors. He has been fully cooked by God.

In this book, you will learn about shaking medicine and how it has been known in various places in the world. We have enjoyed hearing many of these stories from Bradford Keeney, and we know that they hold important lessons and truths. He will also tell you how shaking medicine can be brought into your daily life.

We are very aware that the world is in a dangerous crisis, and there is doubt as to whether human beings will survive much longer. We believe that we have helped hold together the threads and ropes of relationship that enable life to continue. Now, those threads have been weakened by human ignorance, selfishness, and greed. Our greatest hope for survival comes from understanding how shaking medicine can help us revitalize and strengthen the threads and ropes of life.

We grant Bradford Keeney full authority to speak about our healing and religious ways. The Bushman wisdom keepers of the Kalahari bless him to do this work. He is a well-chosen spokesperson for shaking medicine, and we hope that his words will help awaken you to receive the gifts that the gods and ancestors are waiting to give you. We invite you to join us in the heartful shaking that promises to bring the greatest joy and fulfillment into your life. We know that this book can help raise your heart.

IKUNTA BOO
TI!'AE ≠OMA
N!YAE KXAO
GIAO'O KAQECE

G≠AQBA-N!A'AN (HEARTS OF THE SPEARS)
NYAE NYAE CONSERVANCY
NAMIBIA
SEPTEMBER 2006

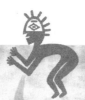

1

THE SHAKE

Rediscovering the Oldest and Newest Cure on Earth

In November of 1881, a Squaxin Indian logger from Puget Sound named John Slocum became sick and soon was pronounced dead. As he lay covered with sheets, friends proceeded to conduct a wake and wait for his wooden coffin to arrive. To everyone's astonishment, he revived in front of them and immediately began to speak, describing an encounter he had had with an angel. The angel told John that God was going to send a new kind of medicine to the Indian people. The angel said the new medicine would not only enable them to heal others, but could also be used to heal oneself without the need of a shaman or doctor.

About a year later, John became sick again. This time, his wife, Mary Slocum, was overcome with despair. When she ran outside to pray and refresh her face with creek water, she felt something enter her from above and flow inside her body. "It felt hot," she recalled, and her body began to tremble and shake. When she ran back inside the house, she spontaneously touched her brother and he immediately started shaking. When she shook over her husband, his health improved the next day. That was when "it came to his mind that this was the new medicine" and that "this medicine was the shake."

From that moment, the Indian Shakers recognized and valued how spiritual inspiration may trigger shaking that leads to a healing encounter.

The Indian Shakers were not the only culture to make this discovery. Shaking bodies and vibrating touch have been known throughout the world as powerful forms of healing expression. Yet the value of trembling, vibrating, quaking, and shaking as a medicine for the body, mind, and soul has been all but lost in recent times, particularly among the more literate and technologically developed cultures.

The purpose of this book is to reintroduce the oldest medicine on earth—the shake. I will examine a number of cultural traditions that practice shaking medicine as a form of healing and highlight the lessons and guidance they bring to us. In addition, a new paradigm for medicine will be presented that includes both arousal and relaxation as necessary co-components for the fullest realization of the healing response. Finally, I will set forth practices that facilitate learning how to shake for therapeutic benefits.

Writing about shaking presents the challenge of describing something that at once is familiar to those who shake but seems bizarre and awkward to understand for those who haven't been seized by this spirited ecstasy of the mind and body. Historically, few shakers have written down their experiences, let alone contextualized them in any theoretical framework. This is partly because shaking medicine has been kept alive in cultures that either lack written language or for whom texts have been given no particular priority. These folks are content to shake, share their ecstatic experiences with their community, and leave it at that.

On the other hand, those with the skills to write who have fallen into the joys and mysteries of the shake may find it difficult to communicate with those who haven't been so moved. There is a fear that they will be disqualified, labeled as having gone off the deep end, having become a cult follower, or, worse, having gone mad. These shakers also keep the shaking to themselves.

For the most part, we are left with brief accounts written by outside observers, usually missionaries or anthropologists who use phrases like "uncontrolled jerks," "spasms," "fits," "convulsions," "shaking frenzy," and "wild movements" to account for what they see. These comments serve as much to describe the observers' bewilderment with conduct outside the familiar grounds of their own experience as they do to describe the experience itself.

For example, the anthropologist Wallace Zane studied shakerism among the "Converted" in the Caribbean island of St. Vincent. His book, *Journeys to the Spiritual Lands,* is a brilliant account of this form of shaking religion. Yet when it comes to one of their most important experiences, shaking, he struggles to understand it. As he writes, "Trying to get at the experience, I asked [the] Converted over and over to help me understand the process of shaking."[1] The words must have been difficult to extract, because his research proceeds to report very little about the experience of shaking.

It wasn't long ago that the practices of Yoga, meditation, and acupuncture were relatively unknown and definitely not mainstream in our culture. Many people feared meditation—and some still do. Psychologists and psychiatrists used the word *xenophobia* (an inappropriate fear of something perceived as foreign or different) to name this unfounded fear. After groups of Western physicians went to China and made public their approval, the quiet practices of the Asian cultures were gradually welcomed to our neighborhoods and universities. Now almost every city and small town in America has someone practicing meditation and receiving acupuncture.

We know, without pausing to doubt, that relaxation and rest help us heal. The idea that relaxation and stillness bring forth healing is a paradigm that Dr. Herbert Benson of Harvard Medical School named the "relaxation response." It is part of the Eastern and Western zeitgeist. What we await is the other half of the picture. The complement to relaxation is arousal. This side of the healing process can be called the "arousal response." What we are ready to learn is that heightened arousal, whether through wild dancing, spontaneous jumping up and down, or body shaking, is as valuable a healing and transformational practice as sitting quietly in a lotus position. This book calls forth the importance of wild activity in our bodies, minds, and souls. As we once let in the healing wisdom of Asia, it is time to let in the healing wisdom of Africa. It is time for the shaking body to become as familiar to us as the quieted body.

I must point out that there are shaking bodies in Asia as well as meditative practices in the African Diaspora. Asia, however, has become a kind of symbol or metaphor for the therapeutic benefits of a stilled body and mind. On the other side of the world, Africa evokes images of heightened body arousal in its ecstatic dances and trembling healers. As I will elaborate in the next chapter, the most powerful form of healing and well-being comes when both hyperarousal and deep relaxation are cycled together, one taking place in relationship to the other. When we shake ourselves to the fullest height of ecstatic expression and then fall into the deepest state of quiet, we set the stage for powerful realignment and evolution of our whole being. This is the whole pattern of holistic medicine.

The next great revolution in medicine, holistic care, well-being, and spiritual practice will be when the practice of shaking is valued as much as the practice of meditation. Joining with my brothers and sisters throughout the world who have kept the shaking traditions alive and well, I invite you to discover the shake. At first it may seem exotic and unnatural. You may have some hesitation and a bit of fear about what seems foreign and radically different from your everyday habits and experience. Remember that the same was true for meditation when it was first brought to the West. But when you experience the shake in its natural form, you will feel that it was always a part of you, an old friend formerly lost but always waiting to be found. We were born to shake, to be fully excited about our aliveness, as we were born to have moments of rest and quiet stillness.

Shaking and quaking have been too easily dismissed by Euro-American scholars (as well as Asian scholars) as being signs of mental distress, neurological disorder, psychopathology, psychological dissociation, or possession by spirits. Shaking is more often assumed to be troubling or evil rather than benevolent. This kind of misunderstanding and culturally ascribed negative connotation has been particularly directed at the more ecstatic religions of Africa. Another way in which the technologically advanced world habitually disqualifies the shaking and quaking body is by dismissing it as an immature stage of spiritual development caused by the overemotionality of the so-called primitive.

There are some authority figures, psychological and clerical, who will sternly advise you to avoid taking any shaking medicine. They will say it hasn't been tested in a laboratory and is a very dangerous substance that can cause mental, physical, and spiritual illness. Some will even say it is a waste of time. All of this was once said about meditation. This criticism is partially right. All things in excess can become harmful—too much water, food, or oxygen will kill you. But the absence of a vital component to life also brings harm.

I must also alert you to the fact that most of us have been taught to be experientially allergic to conduct that appears "out of control." We have cultivated a reverence toward "being in control" and a fear and avoidance of experience that feels "out of control." Most introductory textbooks of psychology even define the profession as "the science of predicting and controlling behavior." The paradox of our time is that the more we try to control ourselves, or others, or our environment, the more out of control everything becomes. Along similar lines, the more we exalt the fantasy of control, the more we seek experiences that provide a moment of letting go, sometimes through sex, drugs, and free expression that pushes the edge of convention. We fail to see the many other, more productive ways of cultivating out-of-control experiences that are necessary to serve the healthy development of our lives, relationships, and ecology.

I propose that this negation of the shaking body constitutes the last great taboo of our time. We have been liberated to do many things with our bodies, from ingesting every imaginable chemical substance, legal and illegal, to stimulating our erotic capacities through endless forms and scenarios. What still remains off-limits, for the most part, is the shake. If you shake, you get psychologically and spiritually diagnosed.

As with all taboos, it's important to remember that no culture is completely successful at eradicating a behavior or social practice. Prohibition eliminated neither the consumption of alcohol nor the bartenders who served the drinks. Drinking went underground, where it continued to thrive. Similarly, when many of the churches and healing traditions all but banned spirited ecstatic expression, it moved into the musical arenas of blues, rock, rave, and techno, not to mention burning-man festivals throughout the world and the sanctified gospel traditions of the African American church. The shaking has never stopped; it is going on out there this very moment, but it usually takes place without any benefit of the collective wisdom that can nurture, deepen, and expand its expression, ripening it into a divine elixir that empowers our presence in everyday life.

For most of the technologically enriched, there is evidence of some kind of starvation. We sometimes refer to this deprivation as spiritual in nature. The malaise and angst that lead to the popularity of spiritual and self-help books, workshops, spas, and well-being centers are traceable to this hunger. Yet the hunger and thirst aren't necessarily being satisfied. Many seekers have become consumers of spirituality, boastfully adding more spiritual experiences, ideas, and habits to their lives. However, journeying to every shaman, guru, rabbi, and priestess in the world and reading every spiritual book seldom bring the joy these people are seeking. Contrast this with the joy found in the life of an African Bushman whose prayer and practice is a shake and a song, whose conversations mention few outside spiritual ideas, and whose entire material possessions can be carried on his or her back.

I am not trying to romanticize Third World spirituality or indigenous lifestyles, but am aiming to draw a distinction that serves to underscore a point: namely, that in spite of the abundance of our material possessions and spiritual knowledge, we are missing something. Becoming more spiritual or more aware of spiritual ideas, stories, teachings, symbols, amulets, paraphernalia, and sayings may not make us more spirited. What we are looking for is spirit rather than spirituality. By *spirit* I don't mean a hypothesized entity or ghostlike presence from another dimension. I am referring to a spirited life, one that is filled with vitality, joy, and occasions of ecstatic delight. "You know you have the spirit when you have the shake." This is the declaration voiced by the world's shakers, from the Kalahari to the Caribbean to the mountains of China and to the African American churches of Louisiana.

Is it then true that if you aren't shaking, you're not happy or fulfilled? I am not saying this. However, if you haven't entered the ecstatic state brought forth by trembling joy, you have missed one of the greatest gifts life presents. Furthermore, once you taste this kind of ecstatic joy, you will want to have it be a steady part of your diet. Perhaps it is better said in the opposite way: Once you feel the biggest joy and delight life has to offer, you will be unable to avoid trembling, quaking, and shaking with happiness.

As celebrated joy lifts our spirit, our body longs to join the party. As delight escalates, our body heads toward the experiential landscape of ecstatic performance. When we enter that domain, our hands and legs start trembling. We feel a vibration come onto our body. Rather than suppress it, we are now free to go further into this moving way of being. Into the shake we fall, sometimes jerking or jumping, shouting or grunting. We enter the healing and transformative experiences of the shaking body. Here we find ourselves, maybe for the first time, in the kindergarten of ecstatic wisdom. We are encouraged to allow the trembling, shaking, and quaking to take over. We experiment with giving up control. This is the entry into shaking medicine.

What is this big joy that makes our bodies shake? Is it the divine bliss of realizing, without distraction, the fact of being alive? What we do know is that this bliss is unconditionally available to everyone on the planet, rich and poor, well and sick, educated and illiterate. It has been referred to as the big love, the grace of God, the great liberation from suffering, the divine light, and the alpha and omega of all that matters to our heart and soul.

Shaking is brought on by divine inspirations and epiphanies. At the same time, shaking can lead to these sacred experiences. Shaking and the holiest experiences are inseparable. In these realms of experience, we are attuned, calibrated, freshly inspired, converted to a mission, infused with spirit, and reborn anew. It is that which we most deeply seek when we feel that something is missing in our lives. It is what some cultures in the world prioritize; they don't let a week go by without the presence of the shake and all the reenergizing and renewal it brings forth. It is their most treasured secret, their fountain of youthful countenance, and their source of vitality. Without it, they would fall into despair and escalating irritability with one another. The shake is their most important truth, their deepest prayer, and their most powerful medicine.

Shaking is the skeleton key that opens the doors to the wild. Whether the Kalahari Bushmen, the Minnesota Ojibway, or the Japanese practitioners of *seiki jutsu*, the followers of each tradition have a system of beliefs and practices that open a portal to a larger experiential universe, a place where vision and imagination run free. This spiritual universe is the place of the wild. This wild space has many names, including "the unconscious," or, as some prefer to expand the term, "the collective unconscious." Here is the realm of systemic webs of infinite patterns of never-ending elaboration and collaboration, as well as the arrows of evolution and devolution. This is the home of the mystic as well as of the old-time naturalist and the new-time shaker.

It is no accident that traditions that seek wild experience also honor the wild in nature. They defend no rigid boundary between the inner wild and the outer wild. Here life becomes fully copresent with death. Into the wild of an ecosystem the shaman goes, fasting for an entry into inner nature. Into the experiential wild the shaman goes, praying for an entry into the truths of the greater ecology. By these ecological truths, I refer to the devoted observation and full sensuous experience of nature in its wild splendor.

The wild is, as Gary Snyder describes it, "elegantly self-disciplined, self-regulating. That's what wilderness is. Nobody has a management plan for it." Wilderness is home to the shamans, Quakers, Gnostics, Taoists, yoginis, anarchists, American Indians, alchemists, Bushmen, Shakers, Sufis, Teilhard de Chardin Catholics, biologists, Druids, Zen Buddhists, and Tibetans, among other ecologically enlightened traditions. It is a world and spirituality that hasn't been reduced to psychological metaphor and explanation. Rather, it maintains a deep respect and awe of the mysteries that are greater than our capacity to understand. This is raw mind and naked wild. In the wild we more readily lose ourselves in order to find ourselves. In this place we trust the wild mind to take care of things. We surrender to its higher authority, higher power, and higher wisdom. In the wild, we are cooked—shaken and baked to become fully integrated parts of the greater community of all living beings.

I never heard about shaking as a child growing up in Smithville, Missouri. But when I was nineteen years of age, I was unexpectedly hit by an experiential lightning bolt and spontaneously began shaking. I have been shaking now for thirty-six years. I don't mean to say that I have been shaking without interruption. I shake every time I feel inspired to do so and find it to be the most important medicine in my life. In my autobiography, *Bushman Shaman: Awakening the Spirit through Ecstatic Dance,* I tell the story of the transforming ecstatic experience that brought forth the shaking. As I walked down a university sidewalk in January of 1971, I felt something very similar to what Mary Slocum experienced in the 1880s. At first, I felt light and calm with a great peace settling in. Within minutes I found a place to sit, and a powerful transformational experience took place.

I felt like a ball of fire became ignited at the bottom of my back. It began to crawl up my spine and send powerful currents of energy throughout my body. That's when the big shake first came on me. As a boy, I had felt gentle trembling, particularly in the emotional country church services led by my father and grandfather, both preachers of the spirited kind. Several times the trembling in a service pulled me into a spiritual epiphany. But that was nothing compared to what happened during that night at the University of Missouri in Columbia. It was my birth as a shaker.

I felt the inner heat, saw the mystical light, and shook all night. Later I found that all the religions of the world have a word for what had happened to me. It didn't matter to me whether it was called satori, mystical illumination, or gnostic transmission. All I knew was that it made my heart open, pouring forth an unrestrained love for all living beings and traditions. There was no exclusion in this rapture of my heart and soul. I knew, without a doubt, that it was the greatest experience a human being could ever have.

From that night on, I was able to shake and quake at will. All I had to do was contemplate inspirational thoughts and the shaking would come. I had to learn to cool down the heat and stop the shaking. At times I even removed myself from spiritual reflection, inspiring music, and spirited events. However, when I shook, I was a wild devotee of the big love. I told no one about my shaking or about my initial experience of transformation. But I went to libraries and bookstores to find books that might tell me more about the secret shaking life I had entered.

The first book I found was *The Evolutionary Energy in Man*, by Gopi Krishna. That's when I was first introduced to the word *kundalini* and the tradition of yoga that nourishes its development. On the one hand, I was thrilled to find out that what had happened to me had been experienced by other people. On the other hand, I felt there was too much theory and verbiage going on in the plethora of yoga texts that I surveyed. I believed that if you had a significant kundalini awakening, you would be less interested in philosophical speculation and instead would want to shake into the divine bliss whenever an opportunity presented itself. Why talk about it when you can be it?

For nearly a decade, I shook only privately. Though I was extremely grateful that the shake had come into my life and believed that it was the greatest gift I would ever receive, trying to find its place in the world frustrated me. Where do I go to shake in public? Whom can I share this with? Can I make a living with the shake? I felt like I had the secret to the universe, but I would sound inflated or crazy if I opened my mouth and articulated the enthusiasm I had for shaking ecstasy.

Fortunately, the shake brought with it an inner voice and guiding force. If I shook and listened, I would be given inner guidance. You can call this enriched intuition, spiritual guidance, ancestral help, divine teaching, God's instruction, channeled directions, or unconscious wisdom. Because it was happening to me with strong authority, I didn't need a name for it. In fact, naming it seemed to be unnecessary and absurd. I simply knew what would happen when I allowed the trembling to tune in to the right frequency or make a connection.

Following this inner guidance, I became a scholar and learned a way of thinking postulated by the systems theorist Gregory Bateson. That, in turn, led me to the work of a number of radical and creative psychotherapists like Carl Whitaker and Milton Erickson. I became an author of books that teach how to know and act in a way that emphasizes systemic patterns and interconnection rather than discrete objects influenced by simplistic causality. As I became a thinker of circular patterns rather than straight lines, I found that I preferred shaking with others rather than shaking by myself. I discovered that I could shake someone just as Mary Slocum could shake others with her trembling hands. Of course, I hadn't heard of the Slocums back then. I was just experimenting with the shaking on my own. To my great fortune, my reputation as a scholar of systemic thinking and therapy led to invitations from various universities and institutes throughout the world. Those trips provided an avenue to find shakers in other cultures with whom I could interact.

I went to the Indian reservations of North America and found medicine people who knew about the shake. I became a part of an inner-city African American church where the spirited expression gave rise to shaking and trembling expression. From there I ventured to the African continent, first invited as a visiting professor and later as a field researcher. Before I knew it, I had assembled a network of notable healers and spiritual leaders whose practice was rooted in shaking medicine.

I also became initiated and recognized as a traditional shaman in various cultures throughout the world. Among the Bushmen I was recognized as a *n|om-kxao,* an owner of spiritual power. In other words, I knew how to shake and administer the shaking medicine. Among the Bushmen I spoke of the Sky God and the trickster gods, while among the Spiritual Baptists of St. Vincent I discussed visionary travel to the spiritual lands through ecstatic movements called '*doption.* In Japan I conversed about *seiki,* their ancient word for the life force, while in the sanctified churches of African Americans I talked about the Holy Ghost that danced us down the aisles. The metaphors and meanings shifted from culture to culture, but the shaking remained the same.

From time to time, I would take a break from my research to speak about these traditions and offer public examples of shaking. I shook in Austin, San Francisco, Chicago, Washington, D.C., New Orleans, New York City, Rio de Janeiro, Johannesburg, Mexico City, Tokyo, and

Lausanne, to name a few places. I published a book series entitled *Profiles of Healing*, described as an encyclopedia of the world's healing traditions. All in all, from the time I first began shaking until the writing of this book, I spent over thirty-six years pondering the mystery of the shaking medicine.

Wherever I went and whatever I wrote, I wondered how shaking could be reintroduced to the contemporary world. Everything I did was understood as a preparation to someday tell the truths about shaking medicine. Even as I was a director of several doctoral programs in family therapy, a distinguished scholar of cultural studies at a foundation, an author of nearly thirty books, and a teacher of numerous classes, workshops, and keynote addresses, the shaking medicine was at the back of my mind and deep in my heart and soul. I found shaking, whether metaphorical or literal, to be the key to personal and relational transformation. The purpose of this book is to share what I have learned with you.

"How can I know more about the shake and learn how to bring it into my daily life? Does anyone shake in my neighborhood? Where do I go to shake? Has the shake become extinct altogether in our culture, or is it an endangered experience? Who else shakes in the world? What can we learn from them? How long will it take for me to start shaking? Are there different kinds of trembling, shaking, and quaking? Do I need a tutor or teacher who can help me shake? What are the lessons learned in shaking? Will my shaking evolve? Will shaking shake up everything in my life?" These are the questions I will address.

What does it feel like when the shake moves you? It is typically not like being put in one of those hardware store machines that shake a can of paint. You probably are not going to get shaken in that kind of violent fashion, although sometimes the ecstatic shaking can whip you around with great vigor. The shake can be gentle or strong. It can be evenly pulsed or it can be syncopated, or polyrhythmic. It can affect a part of your body or the whole of your body. There are as many outcomes and ways of being shaken as there are ways the body can express itself.

When you receive the shake, there are many possible experiences that accompany it. You may experience any of these outcomes:

Highly charged excitement

Simultaneous sense of deep relaxation and heightened arousal

Vibrating, prickling, or tingling sensations; sensations of energy or electricity-like currents circulating throughout the body

Intense heat or cold

Muscle twitches and involuntary body movements: jerking, tremors, quaking, and shaking

Desire to move into an unusual body posture

Awareness of an inner force moving inside you or an inner voice that provides guidance

Feeling of being high ("drunk from the shake")

Intensified sexual desires

Increased heartbeat

Spontaneous emotional expression such as laughing or weeping

Improvised vocalizations

Hearing inner sounds like bees buzzing, drumming, moving water or wind, roaring, whooshing, thunder, ringing, and music

Altered states of consciousness; expanded awareness, trance, or mystical experience

Blissful feelings in the head, particularly the crown area

Pervasive and indescribable ecstatic bliss

Intensified feelings of love, peace, and compassion

Visionary and out-of-body experiences and imagined body flight

Belief that you are acquiring a healing power

Stimulation of the desire for creative expression

Deepened understanding of life; enlightenment, conversion, or transcendent experiences

Any of these experiences can take place when the shaking medicine enters your body. It can happen within seconds or minutes of being shaken. Experienced shakers can sometimes bring about a dramatic impact within ten seconds of the time their trembling hands touch another person. I have witnessed as well as performed this many times. Here's a personal description of how the shake was first experienced by Don Wright, a psychotherapist who attended a demonstration with me in New Mexico. In his words:

> When I hugged him I realized that he was trembling throughout his body. He began to place his hand on my chest, grab and squeeze me, and push me in various ways with an unbelievably high energy. At the same time he was producing strange wind/jungle/animal sounds interspersed with bursts of excited exclamations in an unidentifiable primitive sounding language and in a voice that did not seem to be his own.
>
> I am not sure how long this experience lasted because I seemed to have entered a dream-like state of consciousness, but when he finally stopped I realized that I was extremely energized and vibrantly experiencing myself and everything around me. I felt as if I was almost floating and wanted to move my body with speed and precision. All of my senses were intensified. I recognized this condition as being similar to Ki activation that I had learned to do and utilize in Aikido training. The difference was that the intensity of this energy was magnitudes beyond what I had previously experienced or even imagined could be.

This kind of experience happens on a weekly basis in those communities around the world that are fortunate to have group gatherings of shaking as part of their schedules. Although the entry into shaking medicine is greatly enhanced with the presence of an experienced shaker, there are other ways to bring forth the shake into your life. I will discuss solo practices that can help awaken the shake and present some strategies for bringing relational shaking into your life.

There is no one right way to shake or to learn how to bring shaking medicine into your life. You must experiment, tinker, and try a variety of approaches that aim to awaken your shaking. A faithful commitment to trial-and-error learning will help bring forth the shaking. You can also look for places where shaking is taking place already, such as ecstatic dances and sanctified African American churches. You can allow those social gatherings to get some shaking started in your body.

When you begin trembling and shaking, remember that the first appearance of the shake is like your first day in school. You have the rest of your life to learn more about the vitality, health, transformation, and mystery that shaking medicine can help deliver.

As you enter the shake, you may start asking, "What causes the shake? What makes my body tingle?" Cultures throughout the world have made their own hypotheses and created their own names for what they assume is a force behind the shake. They generally propose that there is a universal life force that we can tap in to, and that its energy brings forth the shaking and all the other energetic outcomes. In China the name for this hypothesized energy is *chi* or *qi*. It is called *ki* in Japan, *n|om* among the Kalahari Bushmen, *tumpinyeri mooroop* among some Aboriginal Australians, *prana* in India, *yesod* by Jewish kabbalists, Holy Spirit by Christians, *baraka* by Sufis, *manitou* by the Ojibway, and *ha* in Hawaii. Among many indigenous people it is simply referred to as "medicine."

It doesn't matter to me what hypothesis or name one believes is the force or cause or pattern behind the spirited expression of our bodies. To argue whether there is a universal life force is to open a never-ending debate. What we can agree upon is that there is such a thing as an aroused, excited body that displays spirited conduct, ranging from tingling to trembling to shaking. Furthermore, we can observe that the aroused body is accompanied by ecstatic experience that is capable of renewing and transforming our lives. I invite you to shake without being concerned about whether it is chi, ki, Holy Spirit, or kundalini. If you happen to believe in one of those notions, then go right ahead and nurture the belief as a way of intensifying the experience. Perhaps you benefit from believing in and using all the different beliefs and names. That is also all right. As they say in Trinidad, particularly among those who belong to as many as five different religions, "The more roads to heaven you take, the better chance you have of getting there." But if any of these names or beliefs distract you from getting on with the shaking, then simply move forward without any attachment to a particular hypothesis and shake for shaking's sake.

In general, we find that whenever the shake is set forth in a culture, the community gathered around its expression has to decide what to do with it. Is it given a positive or negative meaning? Is an institutional structure built around it or is it banned to the margins of the cultural underground? The following chapters discuss how different cultures have tried to give meaning to the shake and how they have managed and orchestrated its expression in social settings. The beliefs that surround the shake contribute to the way the shake is subsequently performed and experienced.

Religious traditions that witness the shake often forbid its unrestrained improvisational performance, demanding that it be controlled through certain practices and ritualistic conduct. In these cases, the meaning of an ecstatic body expression is connoted by the religious authorities, taking advantage of their social position in the religious institution to maintain the hierarchical relations among its members. For Pentecostals, only certain kinds of tremors and shakes are seen as sanctified, while other choreographed movements offer evidence of the need for exorcism. In a different part of the religious world, the practitioners of kundalini yoga in India are also aware of the shake. They assert that kundalini, the name they use to indicate a mysterious force behind the shaking, can get out of control and cause emotional and physical harm. Practitioners must therefore submit to the disciplined teachings of ideological restraints and physical poses to avoid harm and to keep the energy and the social hierarchy under control.

In the Kalahari, one's shaking typically arises in group interaction and is free to dance itself out. Bushman shamans, who arguably know the most about shaking medicine, are easily able to awaken and arouse their bodies to serve the purpose of putting the shake into others. Their trembling hands and bodies touch other people's bodies with the aim of bringing the trembling and the shake into them. To an outsider, transmitting the shake from one person to another may look like a game of tag in which the shake is passed from one body to the next. It surely looked like this when Mary Slocum touched one person after another with her shaking hands and the trembling was found to be contagious. The passing on of the shake is clearly visible when Bushman shamans get together. One shaman passes the shake to another shaman and to anyone else who is open and receptive and appropriately ready to receive it.

It is important to recognize that the person receiving a shake must be willing to be moved by it. If there is resistance, then the shake will not influence. But if there is openness, a readiness for being shaken, the shaman's trembling hands have the ability to transmit the shake. If a Bushman shaman's hands hold your body and the shake comes into you, vibrating you through and through, you may fall into the shaking medicine. In the same way, if your body stands in the sound waves of spirited music and rhythm, you may be moved into the shaking medicine. Or if you simply stand under a tree, a leaf or two may fall and move your body to find the healing pulse, the movement that restores you into wholeness.

A trembling leaf in the wind teaches the trembling hand in a Bushman dance. Both surrender to the elegant wholeness called nature and the minding of its business, which includes our business. When the Zen archer releases the bow, it is the same order of decision made by nature when it decides to drop a leaf off a tree branch. It isn't a purposefully forced drop, and nor is it "not dropped." The dropping is akin to a natural breath moved by the whole that is life. The dropping of the leaf teaches us how to shake. We cannot find the shaking medicine by forcing our bodies to shake. Our shake must be a Zen release of the arrow, a nature-all way of movement.

The mission ahead of you requires a surrender of the attempts both to be still and to be shaken. We must patiently wait to be caught by the medicine. We cannot take this medicine. The medicine waits to take us. It is as if our bodies have invisible strings attached to all our joints. In the hands of a puppeteer, the strings can be pulled and make us dance. We just move with it, not resisting, not anticipating, and never falling out of step with its lead. We face an interesting dilemma. While there is no important knowledge about the shake that can be acquired outside of the shake, we must do everything possible to be ready to be shaken. Our learning is nothing more than a learning to be ready, willing, and able to be moved in a spirited way.

As the Zen teachers sometimes say, teachers can do little more than make the arrangements for an accident. These accidents trip you over your habituated actions and beliefs, stilling things for a moment, and in that moment when the world stops, a breeze waits ready to move you, dance you, and embrace you with the many arms of Shiva's shake. The stories, ideas, and directives of this book aim to help you become ready to be shaken. They both intensify and illuminate your hidden hunger and thirst for a spirited life. They are servants to the shakings, quakings, and tremblings of the gods. All of this is offered, though nothing will be said that hasn't already been said. You are being introduced to the shaking medicine, the oldest and newest cure on Earth.

Years ago, I received a phone call from a woman who was a medical researcher at the Mayo Clinic, in Rochester, Minnesota. She told me about her daughter, a young gymnast who had received knee surgery. She had been an award-winning competitor, but two years after the surgery, she was still unable to compete. Although the best doctors at the Mayo Clinic had worked with her, they were startled to find that after she recovered from surgery, she was unable to perform a forward somersault. She was sent to various clinical departments, from surgery to physical rehabilitation to psychiatry. Among other things, her therapists made her a personalized audiocassette that guided her through some visualization exercises before her gymnastic routine.

No matter what they tried, nothing worked. For two years, she found herself unable to complete her routine. The Mayo Clinic gave up and suggested that perhaps she try an alternative approach, such as hypnosis. The girl's parents subsequently went on a search to find an alternative treatment for their daughter and were given the name of the Milton H. Erickson Foundation in Phoenix, Arizona, a center world renowned for hypnosis and innovative work in psychotherapy. After the director of the foundation listened to her story, he recommended that they have a meeting with me.

When the young gymnast, by now a college student, came to my office, I told her about shaking medicine. I gently shook her knee and taught her a simple exercise that would bring some spontaneous movement into her body. In that first session, her knee began to tingle, and she said that for some unknown reason, she couldn't stop thinking about a special box her grandmother had once given her. I suggested that she be on the lookout for a dream in which she encounters this box. The very next night she dreamed of the box and heard a voice tell her to open it. She did, and found that it held a tiny snake, all coiled up. It didn't frighten her, but it made her curious. We discussed how some cultures depict the snake as a symbol of the force behind the body's ability to tingle, tremble, shake, and move. She was pleased with this idea.

She continued shaking her body, and the dreams continued during the next week. One night she dreamed of being near the edge of a canyon. There she turned into a cloud and was able to fly over the canyon and a nearby forest. I asked her to choose the most important word with which she could remember that dream. She replied, "Cloud," and said that this word captured her feeling of being weightless and able to fly without effort.

In another dream, she saw herself in a gymnastic competition performing her routine with absolute perfection. She chose to name that dream "My Desired Reality," to capture the essence and ecstasy she experienced in it. Together, we constructed a sentence that would capture the dreams that had been brought forth by her shaking practice. The sentence was: "When you see the coiled snake, know that some will see fear, while you see the secret to life, the life force, and shaking energy that turns you into a weightless cloud and effortlessly moves you to your desired reality."

She agreed to carry this sentence with her and to focus on it immediately before performing her gymnastic routine. The very next evening she performed for the first time in three years. She placed in two of her events and led her team to first place.

Shaking medicine has the power to move your body and your dreams. It awakens your body to bring forth the teaching, healing, well-being, and transformation it desires. Although the word *cure* usually refers to remedies and treatments that help make us healthy, it also refers to a transformational process. In the sciences, *cure* means to change the physical, chemical, or electrical properties of a material, doing so through heat, pressure, or catalysts, so as to make the material more stable, durable, and usable. Similarly, when we say that we are cured, we mean that our health has become stronger, more enduring, and more usable in everyday life. Shaking medicine cures us in this regard. It stimulates health and it transforms us to be more capable of full-spirited participation in life.

Sometimes people ask me why their lives have been filled with so much struggle and suffering. I often respond, "Because you are being cured and seasoned to be a fine offering to life's dinner table." I remind them of how fruit, vegetables, and meat are cured and how dishes are seasoned to preserve the finest qualities and enhance the taste. I even mention that the concrete used to make sidewalks and highways must be cured in order for it to be strong, enabling travelers to reach their destination. We go on to discuss how the heat and pressure of suffering are necessary to cure and season us. The greater the pressure and heat of our experience, the more likely we are to become a unique and valuable presence in the world, more able to reach our destiny.

Shaking is the oldest cure. For many of us, it is also the newest cure. Shaking seasons and cures our experience. Whatever has happened to us, both the ups and the downs, can be mixed and shaken, allowing the existential catalytic processes to do their job. I like to say that shaking bodies provide a way in which we "shake and bake" our lives. We need to be baked in order to become risen, resilient, and transformed.

You've heard it said that when the student is ready for the teaching, the perfect teacher arrives. I suggest that the teacher, coach, mentor, or guide you have been waiting for is the leadership of your own body. Ask it to move and direct you. Submit yourself to the ancient way of the shaking wisdom that inspires body, mind, and soul. Join with the many traditions that have honored the importance of the shake. Shake yourself into the life you were born to live.

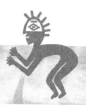

2
THE CYCLE OF HEALING
Ecstatic Arousal and Deep Relaxation

Ecstatic trembling and shaking are the natural expressions of a spirited body. They indicate a process of heightened arousal that contributes to the body's way of bringing forth self-corrective healing, well-being, and transformation. Our past enthusiasm for the therapeutic benefits of stillness, quiet, and relaxation has too often overlooked their complementary partner—the arousal of the mind, body, and soul. Whether through charged physical movement, hyperstimulation, or escalated fervor, human beings can benefit from aroused states of being as much as they do from stable occasions of rest. The next paradigm for healing and medicine will be based upon an awareness and advocacy of the whole cycle of healing—an alternating movement between ecstatic arousal and deep relaxation.

Before setting forth a whole paradigm of healing, let's reexamine the side that is already well known—the practice of meditation and deep relaxation.

Meditation probably began in the original hunter-gatherer societies as people entered into altered states of consciousness while staring at the flames of their fires. Then, over five thousand years ago, the disciplined practice of meditation was described in the Indian scriptures, or tantras. Yoga, which explored the cosmos through inner vision, elaborated on the meditative practice through the use of specialized body postures. Buddha entered the scene around 500 B.C. and became one of the world's greatest proponents of meditation. Other cultures and countries continued to create different forms of understanding and practicing meditation.

In the 1960s and 1970s, the (then) relatively foreign practice of meditation was brought to American soil by the transcendental meditation (TM) movement. Under the leadership of Maharishi Mahesh Yogi, some ten thousand TM practitioners, mostly young people, were inspired to become teachers. Many had first heard of him as a result of his famed influence on the Beatles. To their surprise, they were instructed to cut their long hair, throw away their jeans, and stop taking drugs. It has been argued that by appearing conservative, the movement was able to reach the young people's parents as well. The TM movement's literature convinced even more people to start the practice of meditation. It claimed that meditation was beneficial, easy, fun, and quick. By the mid-1970s, over half a million Americans had learned TM. It was taught in schools, businesses, drug rehabilitation centers, and the armed forces.

TM was marketed to business, academic, and professional communities and had its own university. The teaching of meditation became standardized, beginning with free introductory lectures. If a person decided to sign up for further instruction, he or she went forward with a personal interview and was given a mantra, a specially selected sound or word that was supposed to be kept secret and never spoken aloud. The student was then taught to use the mantra in meditation. The next three teaching sessions took place as group meetings in which students received coaching and more information about the practical details and benefits of meditation. The program was set up to encourage seven progressively advancing states of consciousness, ending with the highest mystical realization that "we are all one and the same."

In 1978, an American legal court decided that TM constituted a religion. Although TM used scientific research to advocate the benefits associated with meditating, it was arguably a thinly disguised version of a Hindu spiritual practice. At about this time, a team of researchers at Stanford University reported that those "who simply relaxed twice daily for fifteen or twenty minutes, using no mantra at all or repeating a mock mantra, found comfort in the experience that did not differ significantly from what the meditators found."[1] The stage was set for medical authorities to take over and define the benefits associated with meditation as natural consequences of the "relaxation response."

The leading voice presenting the efficacy of meditation for health was Dr. Herbert Benson. His research at Harvard University was widely published, and he contributed to such journals as *Scientific American* and the *American Journal of Physiology*. His popular book *The Relaxation Response* led the best-seller lists in the mid-1970s, and is still widely read throughout the world. He showed that meditation brought about physiological outcomes that were the opposite of those brought on by stress. In particular, meditation decreased the heart rate, respiratory rate, blood pressure, oxygen consumption, metabolism, and muscle tension, and slowed down bioelectrical brain waves.

The paradigm set forth by Dr. Benson is based upon not only his research, but also that of the Swiss Nobel laureate Dr. Walter R. Hess. Benson found that the relaxation response brought about by meditation is attributable to two factors: (1) repetition of a word, sound, phrase, prayer, or simple action; and (2) a passive disregard of the everyday thoughts that inevitably enter our minds. He stripped down meditation to its simplest ingredients and proposed a relaxation exercise involving these steps:

1. Select a focus word, short phrase, or prayer based upon your belief system, whether secular or religious (such as "The Lord is my shepherd," "shalom," "peace," "love and light," "enter the stillness," or "deeply relax").
2. Sit comfortably and quietly.
3. Close your eyes.
4. Progressively relax your muscles, starting with your feet, and moving upward to your calves, thighs, abdomen, shoulders, neck, and head.

5. Breathe slowly and naturally. Say your focus word, sound, phrase, or prayer, doing so silently as you exhale.

6. Assume a passive attitude and don't worry about your performance. When thoughts enter, give them no importance and return to your repetition.

7. Continue this for ten to twenty minutes.

8. At the end of the exercise, sit quietly for a moment or two, allowing thoughts to return. Open your eyes and patiently wait another minute before gently standing.

9. Practice the technique one or two times a day, preferably before breakfast and dinner.

Dr. Benson's work was one of many research studies carried out on meditation. Over five hundred papers have been published in over one hundred scientific journals, authored by scientists at over two hundred research institutions and universities, in over twenty countries. Interestingly, Benson's original research subjects were TM practitioners, and they approached him to conduct the research. Benson found that the beneficial effects of using a mantra could be brought forth using words that had nothing to do with Hinduism. He even tried using the phrase "Coca-Cola." His research and popular book demonstrated that some spiritual practices, including meditation or prayer, have clear health benefits regardless of whether their religious proposals are true. He successfully moved meditation from an exclusive spiritual practice to a health care practice. In other words, your health can benefit from prayer and meditation whether or not God exists.

When research convincingly showed improved performance brought about by stress reduction, it wasn't long until one of the world's oldest spiritual practices became a panacea. Today's physicians and medical researchers believe that stress, which triggers the fight-or-flight response, causes or exacerbates a wide variety of medical disorders. The relaxation response, which is the opposite of the fight-or-flight response, is held as effective in helping alleviate and prevent these stress-related disorders. This is subsequently regarded as the physiological basis behind the many mind-body practices that have been historically used to heal hypertension, cardiac conditions, chronic pain, insomnia, anxiety, moderate depression, anger and hostility, irritable bowel syndrome, premenstrual syndrome, and infertility, to mention a few. It is no surprise that over sixty percent of U.S. medical schools teach relaxation techniques. Relaxation therapy is now recommended in standard medical textbooks, and a majority of family practitioners use it in their private practices.

By the 1980s, many corporations and social institutions had a stress-management expert on their staff, and the popular self-help enterprises were proliferating. John Gray, who had been highly involved in the TM movement in the seventies, left to start his own relationship-help offerings. He stopped talking about "flying sutras," a so-called levitation technique taught at the TM Iowa campus, and started talking about men and women from Mars and Venus. Deepak Chopra, an unknown endocrinologist in the mid-1980s, was chosen by Maharishi to head his Ayurvedic medicine program. He left this position to lecture on similar topics under the management of his own teaching business.

Maharishi publicly emphasized that meditation was not a religion, and that people did not have to change their personal beliefs to use it. Because he used the metaphors and authority of science, few could resist deeming his contributions important. Although he frequently used scientific sources to describe the benefits of meditation and sometimes held court with Hans Seyle, the foremost expert on stress at the time, his true aim was never anything less than a spiritual regeneration of the entire world.

In Japan there is an old saying: For every truth, the opposite is also true. This adage points to the natural complementarities that frame our lives, from yin and yang, to left and right, to up and down. For the paradigm of healing, we are reminded that relaxation and arousal are two complementary sides of the whole healing response. Stated differently, health and well-being arise from the interplay of activity and rest. We have long known the benefits of moderate exercise and gentle rest, and with the study of meditation, we recognized the importance of deep stillness and relaxation. Now it is time to examine the place of heightened arousal in the scheme of things related to health.

Practically speaking, we are accustomed to the rejuvenation provided by a good nap or a period of rest. When we are tired, we want to take a time-out. When we feel overstressed, we want to be still and get away from activity. However, there are times when rest and stillness don't help our feeling of being rundown. We may feel low on energy and apathetic about daily life. We feel as if we need an infusion of energy, a revitalization of our body, mind, and spirit. In such times, we require zest rather than rest.

Too much sleep and inactivity can be as harmful as not getting enough. There is an optimal amount of rest and deep relaxation necessary for health and well-being. Similarly, there is an optimal amount of hyperarousal, heightened activity, and ecstatic body expression that serves our optimal state of being. We can benefit from both deep relaxation and ecstatic arousal, regularly administered, to help balance and maintain the homeostasis of our physical being. It is the whole picture of health—the dance between activity and rest, including spirited ecstasy and quiet trance—that requires our attention.

The word *ecstasy* comes from the Greek *ekstasis,* meaning "to be outside oneself." This refers to an exaltation or transformation of ordinary consciousness to a state in which there is a heightened capacity for experience. Synonymous with intense joy and delight, ecstasy suggests emotions so intense that one is carried beyond rational thought and self-control. Ecstasy points to a state of frenzy, rapture, and hyperexcitement. Its opposite is the meditative calm achieved through deep relaxation.

Unfortunately, scholars sometimes reduce their definition of *ecstasy* to that of a trance state, not differentiating the altered states brought about by relaxation from those created by arousal. When discussing shamanic experience, the term *ecstatic experience* is sometimes mistaken for a traditional trance induced by relaxation and guided imagery. As we will see, ecstatic states of consciousness and ecstatic trances are brought forth by arousal, emotional excitement, and behavioral frenzy. For the purpose of this book, we will use the latter definition of ecstasy, applied to both ecstatic experience and ecstatic body expression, to indicate heightened consciousness brought about by hyperarousal.

In villages all over Africa, there are people who go to traditional healers whenever they get sick. Rather than prescribe rest and relaxation, many of these healers will call the community together, bring out the drums, and start dancing around a fire. In the frenzy of an ecstatic dance, bodies will tremble, shake, and quake. Here, healing is brought forth by the experience of shaking medicine. These people believe in the medicinal benefits of supercharged body arousal.

However, if you closely examine an African healing ritual like the Kalahari Bushman healing dance, you find that heightened arousal and deep relaxation are copresent. After someone dances into ecstasy, a climax or plateau is attained, and thereafter the body falls to the ground, entering a deep state of relaxation. What takes place is a full cycle that moves from arousal to relaxation. In an all-night ceremony, a shaking Bushman shaman may experience several of these full cycles.

I propose that this full cycle, in which one climbs toward a high peak of arousal and then falls until hitting a deep bottom of relaxation, comprises a paradigm for the whole healing response. There are significant healing and transformational benefits when we allow our bodies to naturally and effortlessly enter ecstatic realms and then effortlessly shift into deep states of relaxation. Perhaps Africans learned a more effortless entry into the healing cycle by beginning with spontaneous movement. When the ceremonial drums are beaten, the energized rhythms capture the body and move it without effort. One feels danced and shaken by the fervor of the occasion. When the body dances and shakes itself out, it collapses to the ground and enters, without effort, the deep stillness that meditation seeks. This is a non-purposeful, effortless entry into the cycle of healing. Nothing is forced, neither excitation nor stillness.

Scholars of consciousness such as Roland Fischer have been aware of the relationship of hyperaroused ecstatic experiences and hypoaroused meditation. Fischer's work describes two directions in which consciousness can be altered. One direction is called "the ergotropic pathway of increasing arousal culminating at the extreme in mystical ecstasy," while the other direction is "the trophotropic pathway of decreasing arousal resulting in deep meditative trance." Fischer's examination of ecstatic and meditative states allows us to note the physiological correlates of spiritual experience. The ergotropic pathway is physically marked by an increase in the sympathetic nervous system, increased frequency of saccadic movements of the eyes, and an increase in cortical activity. The trophotropic pathway is characterized by an increase in parasympathetic activity, diminished frequency of saccadic movements, muscle relaxation, and decreased cortical activity. Fischer proposes that the farther one moves in either direction, hyper- or hypoarousal, the closer to transformational experience one gets, with the end points of both being the same: an experience described as the oneness or coherent unity of the universe, where there is an experiential absence of distinction and duality.

Fischer's model of consciousness accounts for a phenomenon he calls trophotropic rebound. This refers to passing directly from the height of ecstasy into the deepest state of meditation, sometimes called *samadhi*. Furthermore, the relationship between ergotropic and trophotropic pathways isn't necessarily limited to their extremes. Each level of hyperarousal may have an equivalent rebound level of hypoarousal—what Gellhorn calls "rebound phenomena from the automatic and somatic components of the ergotropic and trophotropic systems."[2] Stated more simply, the degree to which you are intensely aroused is followed by the same degree of relaxation. For a Bushman shaman who dances into maximal ecstasy, the experience will most likely be followed by the deepest experience of meditative trance. In general, the more ecstatic the experience, the deeper and more beneficial the relaxation that follows. It is therefore possible to get to the deepest stages of meditation by going in the opposite direction—via arousal. And we can sometimes get to the highest states of ecstasy through the opposite pathway—via meditative stillness and quiet. Ecstatic and meditative experiences are not separate. The copresence of arousal and relaxation must be acknowledged when we speak of the self-regulating healing processes of the human body, mind, and soul.

Again, as familiar as we are with the practices and benefits of relaxation, we are relatively unfamiliar with the therapeutic practices and benefits of heightened arousal. One example of the latter is found in the work of the Brazilian psychiatrist Dr. David Akstein, in what he calls "terpsichoretrancetherapy." It is a form of trance dance therapy inspired by his study of ritual trances brought on in ecstatic ceremonies, particularly those from the dancing Umbanda cults of Brazil. Terpsichore is the name of the Greek goddess of dance and music. Terpsichoretrancetherapy simply means "dancing trance therapy." It draws upon Dr. Akstein's background as a neuropsychiatrist and scholar of trance in Brazil, a country in which as much as half the population is involved in ritualistic trance.

Years ago, Dr. Akstein was working with a ballet company. He experimentally taught them hypnosis as a way of improving their performance. To his surprise, not only did their dancing improve, but some of them began reporting an improvement or change in their personal lives as well. Soon after, he began experimenting with the use of kinetic trance, the induction or enhancement of an altered state through movement. He had observed how rituals involving highly aroused movements led to trance, and decided to attempt the same outcome with his patients. He took groups of psychiatric patients, played ritualistic music he had recorded, and invited everyone to move spontaneously, dancing in a freely spirited fashion. He found that this kind of trance dancing was a nonverbal group therapy that led to significant improvements in the lives of his patients.

Over the years, he designed a protocol for the movement trance work, which had four components:

1. In the initial preparatory induction, the participants' eyes are closed or blindfolded, and they are instructed to find a singular internal focus while they increase their breathing rate to about forty breaths per minute (panting), tilt their head either forward or backward, and rotate their bodies counterclockwise several times as ecstatic music is introduced. Sometimes, the participants are also instructed to shake their bodies for a while before dancing.

2. At the next stage, the participants move and dance as they wish, doing so for up to forty-five minutes. The dancers have spotters or protectors to shield them from injury and from interfering with other dancers on the floor.

3. Following the spirited dancing, the participants lie down and are made comfortable with relaxing music. This lasts for ten to twenty minutes.

4. Finally, there is a group discussion for the participants to have an opportunity to share their experiences.

Although the therapy is not suitable for people with epilepsy, serious cardiovascular problems, certain motion disorders, and women in the first trimester of pregnancy, it has been successfully used as a treatment for people suffering from a wide range of problems, including most of the so-called psychoneurotic neuroses. The therapy has also proved highly successful as a tool for personal growth and development.

In an attempt to explain the therapeutic benefits of this highly aroused movement therapy, Akstein and Portal propose that ecstatic movement therapy helps bring forth an emotional release:

We have seen the sub-cortical areas are released from inhibition, in particular the limbic system, seat of the emotions. The emotional liberation is maintained by the very stimulating music, facilitating releases, and at the same time preventing them from being totally chaotic forms of expression, by the rhythms, which provides a certain framework.[3]

Observable emotional release is one aspect of the healing process. What is likely happening at a more systemic level is the realignment, recalibration, or tuning of the individual's neurobehavioral organization. The balance, stability, or homeostasis of the whole brain and whole body may be articulated using many different metaphors and theories. However it is specified, as ergotropic-trophotopic tuning,[4] autopoiesis,[5] or the law of cognitive homeostasis,[6] among a few available theories, heightened arousal serves to reset the organization of our whole being. This resetting or tuning applies to all possible levels of biological processes, from neurobiology to behavior to social patterns of interaction. Further scientific research will enable us to advance our understanding of the specific mechanisms underlying hyperarousal's contributions to physiological healing and experiential transformation.

I first met David Akstein in May 1997 at the Evolution of Hypnosis Conference in Brazil. Each of us had been invited to give a keynote address along with renowned hypnotists Ernest Rossi, Betty Alice Erickson, and Jeffrey Zeig. I wasn't familiar with Akstein's work at the time, and after I presented the work I had done with indigenous shamans and their shaking medicine, he ran to the stage and publicly pronounced that I was his "spiritual son." We went off to talk, and he told me about his life and how thrilling it had been to learn from indigenous practices that emphasize ecstatic movements and trance. He also said that his work had been controversial, and that he was criticized for being too involved with marginalized spiritual groups.

He went on to say that many Brazilians, particularly those who were well educated, had double lives. On the public side, they were intellectuals with no professed interest in ecstatic spirituality, but in private, many went to the ceremonies and spiritual advisers of Candomblé, Umbanda, and a variety of other spiritualist groups. It was socially understood that these private lives should be kept secret. Akstein broke the veil of secrecy, and even though his professional work was stripped of any spiritual connotations, the very announcement that ecstatic experience was healthy made him controversial. Akstein, in spite of his medical degree and international reputation, had run into the taboo that hides the shaking and ecstatic sensuous body. He finally left Rio de Janeiro and went to France, where his work continued in the land where Mesmer, one of the early founders of hypnosis, had worked.

Another therapeutic practice that taps into the healing power of shaking medicine is found in the therapeutic work of Peter Levine, who developed a method for treating the symptoms of trauma. Considering ethological observations of animals in the wild, he pondered why animals rarely get traumatized. When a prey animal in the wild is attacked or seriously injured, it has what he calls a "built-in ability to rebound." Specifically, the animals "shake off" the serious attack that threatened their lives. They go somewhere and tremble, shake, pant, take deep breaths, and exhibit rapid eye movements. Free from the language-making of a cerebral cortex, they don't get engaged in language-based therapy and treatment. Wild animals simply allow their reptilian brains to trigger shaking medicine.

One day, while treating a client with anxiety, Levine observed her becoming anxious right in front of him. She could barely speak and was fully panicked. What happened to Levine at that moment forever changed the way he would treat people with trauma. The image of a tiger jumping through the bush flashed in his mind, and he spontaneously shouted at his client, "You are being attacked by a large tiger. See the tiger as it comes at you. Run toward those rocks, climb them, and escape!" His client started to scream, and for almost an hour, she trembled, shook, and sobbed with full-body convulsions. Afterward, she felt "like she had herself again."[7]

What Levine witnessed had been observed for thousands of years by shamans throughout the world and by thousands of bodyworkers in recent times. Namely, the body has a natural way of shaking off its emotional knots. Sometimes a mere touch can trigger such a reaction in the body. Whether the signal takes the form of an imagined tiger or an unexpected touch, the body awaits the signal to shake and quake, to bring forth a healing recalibration of its balance and place in the world.

As I mentioned earlier, not all Asian practices emphasize meditative relaxation, although that is what most Westerners associate with the East. One exception is found in the teachings of Bhagwan Shree Rajneesh in what he called "dynamic meditation." It is similar to Akstein's therapy. Participants begin with deep, fast breathing, and let the body move freely, as desired. This is followed by wild actions that may include jumping, shaking, screaming, and laughing. After ten minutes of this, the participants jump up and down, shouting, "Hoo! Hoo! Hoo!" They do so with the intention of concentrating and compacting energy in their sex centers. After exhaustion, the participants stop and remain in a frozen position, experiencing the energy flowing inside their bodies. This is followed by a celebration of dance and song.

There are many cultural ways of activating aroused ecstasy in the body, including the whirling dance of Sufism, the walking meditation of Buddhism, the ancestral dancing of Shintoism, the ghost dances of the American Indians, and the many ecstatic ceremonies of shamans throughout the world. The Arctic shaman's body shakes, as do the shaking tents of the Ojibway, Cree, and Micmac Indians. Wherever people have sought contact with spirit, shaking was present. One of the original meanings of the word *shaman* actually points to the excited, shaking body of the shaman. The scholar Casanowicz wrote that "the Siberian Tungus word for shaman, *saman,* means one who is excited, moved, or raised." More than anyone, the shamans have been the technicians and masters of ecstatic experience. They are the experts of shaking medicine.

Various Western scholars have observed or read about the ecstatic performances of shamans with the assumption that specific performed actions, rather than the beliefs the shamans profess, are responsible for altered states of consciousness. Michael Harner, for example, peeled away the contextual structure of the shamans he studied, and reduced what he observed to a repetitive thumping of a drum or shaking of a rattle. He declared that it was not necessarily important to have a religious belief, but that entrainment to repetitive auditory stimuli was sufficient to bring about the conditions for a shamanic experience.

Harner called his method "core shamanism," to suggest that he had distilled the oldest shamanic traditions in the world into a step-by-step procedure that could be taught in a workshop session. People first lie down with their eyes closed or covered. A monotonous drumbeat then induces a light trance, setting the stage for what psychologists call a guided imagery exercise. A facilitator guides the group through a fantasized inner journey, suggesting they imagine seeing an entry into the Earth, whether through a cave, a special opening in a tree, or another portal, leading them into a spirit world. There, the facilitator suggests that they find a spirit helper or power animal that can guide and teach them about spirituality and healing. This guided fantasy, called the shamanic journey, is said to help bring forth personal transformation.

Psychotherapists and hypnotists have long used guided imagery that includes animals and imagined helpers to help clients access their inner resources. The sound of a ticking clock or metronome also has been used by hypnotists to induce a light trance, which sets up a more cooperative atmosphere for following the therapist's suggestions for inner exploration. It is no surprise that Harner's shamanic journey yields many of the same benefits found in historically established counseling practices. What he adds, however, are stories, ideas, and metaphors from shamanic traditions that empower the beliefs of people who attend his workshops. The strength of his method may have as much to do with the contextual aspects as with the stripped-down core ingredients of the method.

Harner's teachings become more interesting, from the perspective of arousal-engendering practices, when he discusses the shamanic exercise of "calling the beast," referred to as "a way whereby the people of the community, through dance, evoke or get in touch with their animal aspects."[8] Here, a rattle is first shaken slowly and steadily at about sixty times per minute, while the participants' feet move in the same tempo. With guided instruction, the participants are advised to "sense" (imagine) the presence of an animal, which usually takes place within five minutes. The facilitator encourages people to experience the "emotions" of the animal and to make noises. When this happens, the rattle shaking and movement is escalated to about one hundred shakes per minute, lasting for about four minutes, followed by another increase to one hundred eighty shakes per minute, which is continued for an additional four minutes. After this aroused activity, the participants are instructed to stop dancing and to imagine the animal inside of them. In this shamanic exercise, we see something that looks more like classic shamanism, with an attempt to arouse and move the body into an ecstatic state. It is similar to Akstein's work and other therapeutic arousal strategies, except it adds guided imagery for the participants.

The first comprehensive book on shamanism, *Shamanism: Archaic Techniques of Ecstasy*, written by Mircea Eliade, first defines *shaman-*

ism as a technique of ecstasy. For Eliade, not any ecstasy will do. To be a shaman, he argues, the ecstatic experience is specialized to bring about imagined soul travel. Harner seized the latter part of Eliade's definition, emphasizing imagined inner journeys to a spirit world, but deemphasized the first and arguably most important part of Eliade's definition, which highlights ecstatic experience. Harner teaches sonic-driven light trances that facilitate imagined journeys, whereas Eliade emphasized classic shamanism as involving highly charged ecstatic experiences that could evoke journeys. In the latter, ecstasy is achieved through hyperarousal, typically brought forth by a moving body, not a still body. As Eliade quotes N. V. Pripuzov, "one destined to shamanship begins by being frenzied."[9]

Early scholars assumed shamans were either epileptic or hysterical because of the wild, often convulsive body behavior they witnessed. Eliade proposes that "the only difference between a shaman and an epileptic is that the latter cannot deliberately enter into trance."[10] He goes on to say that "the shamans, for all their apparent likeness to epileptics and hysterics, show proof of a more normal nervous constitution; they achieve a degree of concentration beyond the capacity of the profane; they sustain exhausting efforts; they control their ecstatic movements."[11] Clearly, these shamans have an ecstatic body that is moving.

A perusal of the primary sources of literature on which Eliade based his theories (he wasn't a field researcher) makes it clear that shamans throughout the world shook and trembled, with hyperaroused behavior being the sign of ecstatic experience. For instance, Sieroszewski observed a sixty-year-old shaman who "displayed tireless energy" and "if necessary, he can drum, dance, and jump all night." Similarly, Karjalainen, when describing a Vogul shaman, saw "an energy that appears unbounded," and Castagne watched a shaman who "flings himself in all directions with his eyes shut." He goes on:

[W]ild animal cries and bird calls are heard. . . springing, roaring, leaping; he barks like a dog, sniffs at the audience, lows like an ox, bellows, cries, bleats like a lamb, grunts like a pig, whinnies, coos, imitating with remarkable accuracy the cries of animals, the songs of birds, the sound of their flight, and so on.[12]

Can there be any doubt that the shamanic ecstasy found in cultures throughout the world involves wild behavior and expression? Jochelson found that among the Yukagir, one of the terms to designate the shaman is *'keye,* which literally translates as "the trembling one." Eliade distinguishes between those dressed in shamanic garb who are ritualists and those, with or without costume, who are ecstatics. Dave Gehue, a Micmac medicine man, once told me, "No shake, no shaman." Shamans are the performers of ecstasy, and they show it with a shaking body. You know when you have stepped into ecstatic experience because you look and feel intoxicated when it is over. After taking the shaking medicine, your pupils are widely dilated, it is difficult to walk a straight line, and you feel extremely high. Eliade also acknowledges that the feeling of being drunk and radically disoriented after a spirited ceremony "is the well-known sign of a genuine ecstatic experience."[13]

Another anthropologist, Felicitas Goodman, also stripped away ancient contexts of spiritual performance in an attempt to reveal its bare bones. After she conducted fieldwork in the Yucatán, where she observed ecstatic experience and trance in some charismatic apostolic churches, her students wanted to know what the spiritual experience was like. At first she ignored ecstatic behavior and focused on trying to induce a religious-like trance. Rather than have the students sing hymns of praise, she had them focus on their breath. She believed that church singing primarily served to focus attention, a prerequisite of trance. She didn't notice or didn't emphasize that it was also a heart-centered means of excitation. Therefore, she chose to have her students follow a simple meditative method of concentration and focus. Similarly, instead of clapping hands, which she had seen in the churches, she introduced the rhythm of a shaking rattle (at two hundred ten beats per minute). Her outcomes were disappointing, and she suspended her investigation.

Later she was reinspired by the research of psychologist V. F. Emerson, who suggested that physiological changes result from different body postures used in meditation. She then experimented with inducing non-ordinary states of consciousness by having her students assume the postures portrayed in ancient depictions of spiritual practice and shamans. Her hypothesis was that "certain works of non-Western art—such as figurines and rock paintings—are not simply expressions of creativity, but in fact are ritual instructions."[14] She believed that if you sit like a shaman, you increase the chances of getting a shamanic experience. To a skilled clinical hypnotist, it is not surprising that specified postures, along with any accompanying lore and images about their historical origin or spiritual association, provide contextual cues for the indirect hypnotic suggestion of particular forms of experience. For example, if you stand with your arms reaching toward the sky, it is more likely that you will fantasize flying or ascending into the heavens. Add a drawing of a deeply entranced goddess reaching for the sky, and the persuasive effect is further enhanced.

When the postures were done with the beat of a shaking rattle, or with her later inclusion of dance, they enhanced the outcomes. Like Harner, Goodman observed that bringing more of the shamanic context into the practice enhanced the work. She also noticed that her students, particularly if they were in a standing position, sometimes trembled and shook. After years of experimenting with induced trance experience, her colleague Belinda Gore concluded that "without the opportunity to regularly alter our bodies and our consciousness in a religious trance, we experience what Dr. Goodman calls 'ecstasy deprivation.'" They, too, were aware that ecstatic experience is a vital component of human health and well-being.

The psychiatrist Dr. Stanislav Grof, another pioneer of consciousness research, developed the technique of holotrophic therapy with his wife, Christina Grof. They focused on using hyperventilation brought on by accelerated breathing to induce non-ordinary states of consciousness. The Grofs' work is based upon the observation that intense breathing is seen in "various shamanic procedures, aboriginal healing ceremonies, the healing dance of the !Kung Bushmen and other groups . . . and for different spiritual practices." Using music, holotrophic breathing often brings forth heightened body arousal. These methods are similar to the intentional hyperventilation practices used in siddha yoga and kundalini yoga, and the Grofs noted that kundalini energy could be activated, resulting in an ecstatic display of body shaking and movement.

In this work, the Grofs observe: "In most instances, the breathing experience follows an orgiastic curve, with a build-up of emotions and physical manifestations, culmination, and more or less sudden resolution. . . . At this time, the breathing can actually be extremely slow."[15] What he observed is the whole healing cycle, moving from heightened arousal to deep relaxation. Dr. Grof wisely advises that the facilitators of holotrophic therapy not intervene at all when this change takes place. He encourages the body rhythm to follow its own course.

There has been an ever-expanding proliferation of therapies and practices throughout the world that have noticed the healing and transformational response brought forth by heightened body arousal. Some, like those previously discussed, begin by trying to identify the most basic action or sequence of actions that underlie the efficacy of ancient shamanic and ecstatic religious practices. It is not surprising that Western anthropologists and investigators have sought to reduce a spirited context to an underlying action responsible for a unique outcome. It is the same strategy used by a pharmacology researcher who collects indigenous plants and ships them to a biochemical laboratory to identify the chemical compound responsible for the medicinal effect. The pharmacological corporations and the investigators of shamanic experience employ the same strategy: reduce the context to a basic ingredient that can then be solely administered to bring about the desired outcome without the complexities of the original contextual structure. Herbert Benson did the same when he reduced the spiritual practice of meditation to a simple relaxation procedure.

Note that there is sometimes not only a screening to find the activating agent, but also a reduction in what is determined to be the desired outcome. For instance, Harner, following the historian of religion Eliade, chooses the experience of imaginary travel as the most important aspect of shamanic experience. Other aspects of shamanic experience are either ignored or made less important. Similarly, Benson reduces the desired outcome to the relaxation response, ignoring the goals of spiritual development originally posed by meditation practitioners.

However, having made these reductions, researchers later find that their work is enhanced if they bring in more and more ingredients of the whole context. The room may be filled with spiritual context markers such as smoking sage, music, and spoken stories about shamanic cultures, which serve to enrich the context. Additional physical movement, shaking, and dancing may be added to further empower the rituals.

In the case of Herbert Benson, a special word or phrase was added to make the relaxation response more effective, though he avoided calling the phrase a mantra. Benson even went on to write another book, *Beyond the Relaxation Response,* which argued that "the Faith Factor"—that is, bringing in one's beliefs—enhances the relaxation response. It seems reasonable to assume that it will be beneficial to continue examining what has been left out of the contexts these investigators originally studied. In this way, we may find more clues about how to further enrich and empower our contexts of healing.

I have spent more than a decade working with shamans throughout the world and have, at their request, helped them voice their own words and ideas about their practices (see *Profiles of Healing* book series). Sometimes, out of curiosity, I tell them what anthropologists and psychologists have written about their ways. They are usually very pleased that others are interested in their culture and want the world to know about them, but it is not unusual for them to fall to the ground laughing when they hear how their healing practices have been reduced to simple techniques and understandings. They aren't upset, but are bewildered as to why anyone could miss what they regard as most essential. For many of them, it is their love of a Big God, their sacred songs, or the long ordeal of preparation for ecstasy that matters most, not the simple actions of escalated breathing, steady drumming, or special postures. They surprisingly say that the techniques the anthropologists emphasize aren't always needed to activate the ecstatic experiences that heal and transform. "You breathe that way because thinking about your ancestors makes you excited and happy." "We play the drum because we are full of spirit." "I sit that way because I am tired of dancing." These are the kind of responses I have heard.

I don't want to dishonor or make light of the contributions Western scholarship and its method of efficient reductionism provide. My present purpose is to note that Western scholars look at a context and attempt to reduce it to a singular action or magic bullet, whereas indigenous cultures work in the other direction. They strive to build and maintain the whole integrity of their context, underscoring and respecting its complexity and mystery. They often go further and continuously elaborate the interwoven complexities of their healing contexts. To say that what is essential about their context is reducible to rhythm, posture, or respiration is absurd to them. Perhaps it's the same absurdity Western investigators would feel if they were told that the studied outcomes are brought about by one drumbeat or one inhalation. Such a reduction isn't believable because it strips away too much of the patterned sequence of other beats and breaths.

Nevertheless, researchers, therapists, and consciousness explorers often come to the same conclusion, however they are theoretically pronounced. After their initial efforts to bring forth healing responses with minimal action, they start tinkering with ways to enhance the work. Piece by piece, more of the original context is brought back. Perhaps it's time to consider that context is the single most important ingredient. This is the challenge of the contemporary medical scientist, anthropologist, healer, therapist, and physician: in addition to reducing a cure to its most active ingredient, we must consider how to rebuild the context to enhance its effect.

We may find that it is as important to consider the context within which a pill is ingested as it is to ensure the chemical potency of the medication. Imagine being prescribed a CD of music and spoken words or a DVD of a dramatized ritual that helps construct a mood or a mindset—that is, a context for taking your meds. The ancient shaman may come back again, not only to bring us the medicinal plants, but also to introduce us to the songs, images, and movements that construct a context for administrating the plant. Holistic medicine must address more than whole mind–body systems. It must reestablish the importance of the whole contexts that constitute the homes of our experience.

With this recognition of the need for a more whole holistic medicine, I want to return to the proposal that a paradigm of healing must include the natural cycle that swings between ecstatic arousal and meditative relaxation. I earlier argued that we must now include the arousal response as well as the relaxation response. Our examples of a variety of arousal-based therapies, based largely on shamanic and spiritual practices, show that they are very similar. A reversal of Benson's prescription for evoking the relaxation response leaves us with a mirror image that loosely identifies the common ingredients of the arousal response:

1. Focus on good feelings, preferably love, compassion, and kindness, and stay connected to them. It doesn't matter what words or phrases, if any, come to mind.

2. Turn on some spirited rhythmic music and start wiggling and moving.

3. It doesn't matter whether your eyes are open, half-closed, or closed. Allow them to be in whatever position feels natural.

4. Activate your muscles, wiggling and moving them from head to toe.

5. Gradually increase the rate of breath until you are breathing rapidly.

6. Assume an active attitude toward becoming excitable; encourage yourself to tremble, shake, and quake.

7. Continue for as long as you wish.

8. At the end of the exercise, let your body do what it wants—lie down, sit, walk, or whatever feels right.

9. Do this when you desire, even once a day, but at least once a week.

The above steps can be modified in many ways, but they demonstrate that the general way of bringing forth arousal is to do the opposite of what is prescribed for the relaxation response. As with the bare bones of Benson's prescription, know that building up more flesh and context to the prescription for the arousal response will enrich and enhance its effect.

Now we have both a prescription for the relaxation response and a prescription for the arousal response. Immediate questions arise: How does a person who recognizes the importance of both arousal and relaxation maintain optimal health? Is it important to practice both meditation and ecstatic ritual? Would it be wise to practice the relaxation response in the morning and the arousal response in the afternoon? Is it the case that some people are more inclined to work with relaxation rather than arousal and vice versa? Do we need to listen to what our body desires for any given day? This is new ground for exploration. In the forthcoming chapters, we will see how other cultures have addressed these questions. We will also explore new ways of weaving the whole healing cycle into our lives. And we will explore how to add flesh to the bare bones of these approaches, bringing forth more context and vitality.

The first doctors on Earth, the shamans, often observed how animals took care of themselves. They watched how animals would stretch out, and then at the final moment, they would vibrate and shake.[16] Shamans noted that throughout the animal kingdom, creatures spontaneously trembled, shook, and quaked. It appeared to be one of the ways animals kept themselves fit, adjusted, and ready for the next dramatic enactment of life. It should be no surprise that the people with the world's oldest enduring culture, the Kalahari Bushmen, whose lives and beliefs are built upon what they observe in nature, turn to trembling and shaking as their most important medicine. We will look at what they have learned about shaking medicine and discover what it can teach us.

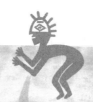

3

THE WORLD'S FIRST SHAKERS

The Kalahari Bushman Shamans

The world's oldest living culture, that of the Kalahari Bushmen, most likely holds the oldest healing practice on Earth. It is based upon a disciplined way of arousing and orchestrating ecstatic body experience. Bushman shamans are masters of spirited expression. They know how to initiate body shaking and use the shake as a medicine when they touch others. Arguably more than any other culture, the Bushman culture has explored and fine-tuned this kind of healing. Over the course of a decade I was initiated into their way of shaking, which emphasizes a vibrant form of healing touch. I will share what I have learned about the Bushman practice of shaking medicine.

The story of how I became a Bushman shaman—beginning as an initiate and ultimately becoming an elder who teaches other Bushmen about the shaking medicine—is set forth in my autobiographical work, *Bushman Shaman: Awakening the Spirit through Ecstatic Dance.* I kept this information to myself for many years, but as I began to write about the Bushmen's spirituality and healing practices, anthropologists and scholars wondered how I had acquired knowledge about their experiential world. Although the Bushmen had been intensely studied by numerous scholars over many years, including members of the Harvard Kalahari Research Project, some of the more essential aspects of their healing ways had been misunderstood or missed. I finally went public and began telling a few well-known scholars about how I came to know the Bushman practice of shaking medicine: I knew about their shamanism because I had become one of their shamans.

One of the first scholars I shared this with was the distinguished rock-art scientist Professor David Lewis-Williams. He had founded the Rock Art Research Laboratory at the University of Witwatersrand in Johannesburg, South Africa. One of the most respected rock-art scientists of Africa, he advanced the shamanistic hypothesis of rock art. He argued that rock art was usually the rendering of a shaman's ecstatic experiences and altered states of consciousness. He based his theories on historic ethnographic reports about Bushman shamans and the scientific literature regarding how human beings enter into and experience altered states of consciousness. Being in southern Africa, he had access to Bushman rock art, and my fieldwork with the Bushmen was of interest to him.

When I presented my data to the professor, he was thrilled to see how it further confirmed the idea that Bushman rock-art images often depict the Bushman shamans' experiences in their healing dances. Over the years, we developed a cordial friendship. I would meet with him after I had been out in the African bush and discuss my latest findings and experiences. I also met with the other scholars of the Rock Art Research Institute, and we examined rock-art images and discussed Bushman shamanism.

On one occasion, the senior scientists of the institute went out into the field with me, and I introduced them to some of the Bushman shamans. Keep in mind that all of these scholars were professed atheists who declared that they personally dismissed spiritual beliefs. Their relationship to me was complicated by my assertion that the Bushmen's experiences were something other than hallucinations. I would say to them around an evening campfire in the Kalahari, "How is it possible for me to dream one of their important dreams if no one has ever written or spoken about it?" I knew they could not understand that some shamanistic experiences are not explainable. From their belief system and point of view, I too must be hallucinating, and surely the Bushmen were simply being polite and placating me by saying I had dreamed something important. To test their hypothesis, one of the scientists told some Bushman shamans the next morning that he had had a special dream about a zebra. He made up what he was saying, expecting to prove that the Bushmen had been placating me over the years. To his surprise, they looked at him as if he was crazy and said they didn't know what he was talking about.

Later in the day, when the rock-art scientists were napping, the Bushmen took me aside and asked if these men were troubled or confused. They were teasing, but at the same time, they sincerely didn't understand why the scientists didn't get the essence of their healing way. They had become used to anthropologists asking them odd questions, and told me they didn't believe it was possible for some people to understand. In their words, "[y]ou must have the right feeling in your heart to understand us." On my part, I sincerely appreciated my friendship with my scientific colleagues (and they remain my close colleagues) because they helped me understand how well-educated and well-intentioned outsiders would react to reports about shamanic experiences.

I learned firsthand that there is an experiential universe that the Bushman shamans are able to enter, and it is opened by the shaking medicine. One of the major discussions I had with the rock-art scientists over the years concerned my discovery that some of the previous anthropological work conducted by eminent scholars was incomplete and at times off the mark. They countered by persistently asking me to specify how the other scholars' work could be mistaken.

The gist of the matter was that some of the earliest ethnographic reports proposed that the Bushmen believe their shamans primarily engage in a battle with the ancestral spirits *(g‖auansi)*, whom they regard as the cause of disease. More recently, in an article entitled "At War with God: Ju‖'hoan Curing Dances," Jan Platvoet, a scholar from Leiden University, proposed that "God and the deceased were blamed [by the Bushmen] for the evil present in the group, were declared personae non gratae and refused admission to the dances as unwelcome aliens . . . [as they] waged a continual ritual war upon them as their sole enemies."[1] Here the mood of a shaman is dramatically depicted as that of a warrior battling God and malevolent ancestral spirits. Practically all descriptions of Bushman healing have been framed this way.

I found the opposite—namely, that the shaman's mood was filled with great love for the ancestors, especially for those loved ones from their own families who had passed on. The Bushman people longed for their missing ancestors' presence and pleaded with them to help cure the sick and renew the community's well-being. Sometimes the ancestors made them feel a little sick so they would be reminded to shake and take care of themselves. And sometimes deceased ancestors would miss their loved ones on earth so much that they wished those living would pass over and join them for company. But the loved ancestors were largely benevolent, and the imagined interactions with them were love-centered. (For a detailed explanation of the Bushman religion, written by Bushman shamans themselves, see the afterword.)

There were other presences that could inflict harm, like previous shamans who had been more interested in being manipulators of power than in healing. However, in general, people were usually made sick by bad feelings (anger, jealousy, arrogance, and selfishness), whether they came from living relatives or dead ones. In addition, the shamans told me that another reason people become sick is that they don't dance enough—that is, they don't receive enough shaking medicine. Whatever the cause of illness, the loved ancestral spirits were usually there to help and empower the healing.

"No, that is not possible!" my colleagues would exclaim. "How could so many scholars have gotten it wrong?" Their questions reminded me of a story my high school science teacher, Robert Sandquist, once told me. Some time ago, there was a woman who cooked the best ham anyone had ever tasted. When asked by a famous chef what her secret was, she said the only thing she knew that was radically different about her preparation was that she cut off the end of the ham before she cooked it. She explained that her mother had taught her this method. Her mother, sitting by her side, agreed and said that this was how *her* mother had always cooked it. At the next holiday dinner, the daughter and mother were pleased to tell Grandmother that a renowned chef was interested in how the family made their special ham. They told her how they assumed the secret must be cutting off the end. Grandmother started laughing and could not stop. Finally, when she got hold of herself, she said, "But my dears, I only had to cut off the end because I had a small cooking pan."

The moral of this story is that sometimes a person starts an idea or a practice and then everyone subsequently follows it without questioning whether it is meaningful or true. In the case of the anthropological study of the Bushmen, the earliest scholars had recorded several ideas about healing that were likely misunderstood or set forth by inexperienced shamans. There are clues that the latter might be the case: some shamans in the earliest interviews described themselves as not being the strongest shamans and not yet capable of the most important shamanic experiences.[2] One of the Bushmen interviewed by the John Marshall expedition, |Kunta Boo, of Tsumkwe, Namibia, told me that the first white people the Bushmen met (the Marshall family) didn't interview their strongest shamans because they conducted their interviews during the day when the shamans were out hunting. Future anthropological work presumably made the assumption that the early reports were accurate, so they kept quoting them as the authoritative sources. The incomplete view of Bushman healing was repeated, article after article, book after book, through the years.

I don't want to be too harsh on previous anthropological work. Many anthropologists have made remarkable contributions to our understanding of Bushman life, and all in all, the mistakes weren't indicative of having been misled or using faulty interview techniques. It was more a matter of not having the complete picture, assuming that one description was the whole rather than a part. For instance, the Bushmen do believe that the occasional bad feelings of living relatives and dead ancestors can make them sick while the largely benevolent ancestors can also make them sick as a means of helping them remember to practice their way of well-being rather than making mischief or stalking them to make a kill.

I began my work with the Bushmen when I was a university professor researching and teaching the nature of personal and social change in a therapeutic context. I had followed the footsteps of my mentor, anthropologist Gregory Bateson, who tried to articulate a systemic view of mind and relationships that was a radical alternative to traditional psychological and sociological explanatory metaphors. Whereas an academic trained in clinical psychology (or an anthropologist turning to psychological ideas) would be more inclined to give the Bushmen psychological tests and structured interviews, my background emphasized interactive knowing, the kind of participatory engagement that is more akin to the conduct of an improvisational actor than to a social scientist armed with theories and instruments. Whereas most social scientists believed that "in order to act, you must first understand" (give tests and ask questions), my axiom, following an interactional perspective, was "In order to understand, you must first interact." From my orientation, to understand the Bushmen's shaking and dancing I had to first dance with the Bushmen and continue dancing with them (rather than emphasize interviewing them). This interactional and improvisational way of participating was familiar ground to the profession of interactional psychotherapy, which I taught and practiced in both university and clinical settings.

The turning point in my interaction with scholars came when I met one of the members of the Harvard Kalahari Research Project who was also cofounder of the Kalahari People's Fund, the superb anthropologist and folklorist Megan Biesele. She was one of the most respected scholars of Bushman culture and was a dedicated advocate of the Kalahari people. It was a priority of hers to make sure they were understood with respect, clarity, and accuracy.

Although we had never met, I invited her to come to my house and review my findings. At the time, I lived in Tucson. The day before Megan arrived, my wife discovered some peach-faced lovebirds in our backyard. They were indigenous to Namibia, where both Megan and I had studied the Bushmen. But, as my wife found out from the Audubon Society, they had over the years become a feral species in Phoenix, though they were rarely sighted in Tucson. It seemed quite an omen for the birds to show up the day before Megan's visit.

During her visit, Megan said she was familiar with the dreaming that can take place in the Kalahari. She too had experienced dreams there that helped advance her understanding of Bushman folklore. Furthermore, she accepted the power and truth of their shaking medicine. She had experienced firsthand how it heals and transforms. Most importantly, she acknowledged that not all of the anthropological data had been published. She proposed that my work did not contradict the whole of what anthropologists had found, but that some scholars had published only a portion of it—the part that made sense to them, that fit within their coherent theory as to what was going on.

After our visit, Megan went back to Africa and interviewed some of the shamans I had worked with. She then graciously endorsed my work:

> There is no question in the minds of the Bushman healers that Keeney's strength and purpose are coterminous with theirs. I know this from talking myself with some of the Kalahari shamans who danced with him. They affirmed his powers as a healer and their enjoyment of dancing with him. . . . He knows whereof he writes, having traveled "ropes to God" himself for much of his life, in many places in addition to the Kalahari.[3]

The key to the anthropologists' confusion was that they misunderstood what they regarded as incoherent discourse among the Bushmen. Most of them overlooked that the Bushmen have a different kind of coherence and logic. Bushmen don't put their thoughts together or see the world in the same way as anthropologists. The Bushmen knew this discrepancy and had a nickname for anthropologists. Behind their backs, they called them the "line people" *(!huijuasi)* because they consistently saw things in terms of simple lines ("this leads to that") and were blind to circularity ("everything is connected to/woven with everything") and the never-ending process of change that underlies all of life.

To the Bushmen, everything in life changes and shifts form, from the climate of the ecosystem to the climate of our personal emotions. This ever-changing universe implies that our words, ideas, and beliefs also keep changing. In fact, one of their most important words is *n!o'an-kal'ae*, referring to the changing force behind the creation of all things, good or bad. Even their understanding of God has two aspects: a relatively stable meaning of the Sky God and the shape-shifting trickster aspect of God, the never-stable form that changes identities and intentions without notice. With the Bushmen's shape-shifting cognitive world of words, meanings, and theories sympathetic to the shifting manifestations of nature, it's no wonder an anthropologist would be confused. The Bushmen's word for God is different one day than it was a year earlier. Sometimes they might say, "The ancestors want to make us sick," and other times they say, "The ancestors love us and they would never want to hurt us."

Anthropologists and Western scholars, with some exceptions, participate in intellectual traditions that revere stable, consistent, and coherent theoretical constructions. When the Bushmen's utterances can't be fit into what the anthropologists regard as a consistent theoretical frame, the scholar is prone to declare things such as "the belief patterns of Bushmen . . . [are] multifarious, inchoate, and amorphous . . . [and] seem to be a confusing tangle of ideas and beliefs, marked by contradictions, inconsistencies, vagueness, and lack of cultural-wide standardization."[4]

Bushmen see the constant changing of forms, or shape shifting, taking place everywhere they look and listen. Plants start as seeds and become sprouts, roots, stalks, and blossoms. Weak infants become strong adults and end up as weak elders. Saltpans and riverbeds are dry one month and wet the next. Their emotions may be sad and complacent one moment but happy and jubilant later on. Even their healing dance starts as a light-hearted gathering, filled with teasing, only to turn to the serious business of shaking medicine, followed by a return to levity.

If both inner and outer natures are always changing, then words, meanings, and explanations must also change to match what is experienced in the world. That is the key to understanding how Bushman elder shamans cognitively put the world together. To Bushmen, it is those anthropologists, with their simple ideas of how understandings should be stable in a single, fixed way, who are often out of tune, out of step, and out of connection with the more dynamic ways of the natural world. Once anthropologists shift their ways of knowing and expressing toward a view of circularity and dynamic transformation,[5] the Bushmen's world appears systemically coherent and consistent.

It should be no surprise that shaking is the most important experience to people who understand the shape-shifting quality of the natural world. Shaking is an enactment and body metaphor of *n!o'an-kal'ae*, the force that keeps changing everything. It is the live performance of an ever-shifting, altering, transforming world. Shaking medicine, from this perspective, helps the human being loosen any over-attachment to a form, internal or external, that is in need of release. It is a Kalahari version of the dance of Shiva, which throws us into the belly of creation and destruction, of life and death.

How can we relate to the force, the energy, or the dynamic that keeps things moving and changing? How is it experienced and how can it be tapped for beneficial effects? The Bushmen refer to the presence of what they call *n|om*. It is believed to permeate the living universe and arises from the changing force of creation, that which makes and keeps things alive. It is similar to what others call the universal life force, chi, ki, kundalini, or the Holy Spirit, among other names.

For the Bushmen, shaking is brought about by *n|om*. Keep in mind that no Bushmen seriously analyze *n|om* or painstakingly hypothesize over what it is or how it brings about energetic displays. I believe they would be just as content to say, "Shaking is brought forth by 'that which shakes us.'" To them, it is more important to know that when the body is deeply aroused or emotionally touched, the body shakes. They appreciate that the deepest and most meaningful arousal of the body, mind, and soul arises from the feelings we have toward those we dearly love. Surely, you can imagine trembling or shaking from being filled with pride, power, or erotic excitement, but these feelings are nothing compared to the remarkable love one can feel for one's children, grandchildren, parents, or grandparents. The biggest love one can imagine and experience brings on the most important trembling, quaking, and shaking.

It could be said that shaking is a love medicine for the Bushmen. When they feel an overwhelming love for family, community, nature, and the Sky God, the seismic activity gets high, strong enough to transform their consciousness. In the beginning stage of becoming a shaman, a Bushman may experience only power and not be able to access the deeper transformation that the shaking based on intense love brings forth. This is part of the shaman's training. Bushman shamans learn not only to shake, but also to direct the shake toward diverse forms of inspiration, expression, and transformation.

Every part of the body can learn to tremble, including hands, arms, feet, legs, belly, torso, and head. Once the shaman becomes comfortable with all the ways of being shaken, the next learning is ready to take place. For Bushman shamans, the shaking must become concentrated in the belly, where a strong feeling of vibrating tightness is brought forth. It becomes so tight that the shaman often feels heat and some pain. If the shaking is concentrated in the belly, a body movement that feels like an internal pump will start. The body feels like it has an internal piston pumping from the abdomen all the way up the chest—raising the energy from the belly to the heart. This pump, which moves raw power toward heart-centered love, sets the next stage of working with the shaking medicine.

As a shaman becomes familiar with the pump, allowing it to move up and down while stomping the feet in the healing dance, the pulsing energy becomes concentrated and directed by this up-and-down movement. Soon the tremors are pumped into the mouth, where sounds are spontaneously generated. At first, the sounds may be noises of the wild, such as those of shamans throughout the world described by early ethnographers—screams, grunts, howls, barks, bird calls, and other unidentifiable noises. With practice and acquired familiarity, the sounds transform into a rhythmic performance. The sound is like the human voice imitating drums. It is interesting to speculate whether this experience—ecstatic rhythms being pumped up the body in a shaking performance of ecstasy—was the originating source of African drumming.

As the body trembles, quakes, shakes, and pumps in synch with the energized voicing of rhythm, the person in training is recognized by other Bushmen as someone who is becoming a shaman. This is the dance that holds transformational efficacy, distinguishable from the beautiful choreography around the fire familiar to anthropologists and tourists. This dance, the alternating stomp of a shaman who is pumping ecstatic energy up his or her chest, is the shaman's dance. In this experiential realm, the dancer must hold on and not topple over and succumb to the temptation to pass out. The initiates believe they are invulnerable to harm. They must not be distracted by the urge to stand on their heads in the middle of the fire, challenge any enemy to take them on, or run wild into the dangerous bush, where lions may be waiting for dinner. More experienced shamans and members of the community try to protect these beginning shamans from hurting themselves. Learning to be comfortable with the shaking and then learning how to bring on the pump may take years of practice with hands-on assistance from more experienced practitioners. Even more experience and training is needed to learn how to keep pumping while deepening the ecstatic movements and releasing the rhythms in a natural and effortless manner.

As a shaman continues learning to shake and pump, allowing the ecstasy to boil, more experiential transformations may take place. The shaman may begin to see, hear, smell, or feel the drawing of his hands toward someone who requires some shaking touch. This is when the doctoring takes place. The shaking medicine is administered by applying shaking hands, arms, and bodies to other people's bodies. The shake is passed into others. For those ready to be shaken, they too will start shaking. Bushmen believe that those who don't shake when touched in this vibrant way still receive the benefits of shaking medicine, although they aren't yet ready to fully receive the shake.

When they see a person start to feel a cramp in the body after receiving a shake, or see the person start to tremble, Bushmen say that a shaman has given that person an arrow, thorn, needle, or nail. This object is how they see the shake entering another person's body. One of their explanations goes like this: In the beginning of time, the Sky God created the world and all the living beings on it. Wanting to express love to this creation, God sent a song to each living being. The honeybee, giraffe, elephant, and every other living creature received a song, which was God's way of delivering love. To send the song, an arrow or thorn was used to throw it through the air and into the body of the recipient.

Imagine God making an arrow, fully concentrating on the big love felt for all creation, trembling with ecstasy. Bending over, singing forth, God squeezes the big love into a narrow arrow or thorn so it can be delivered as a gift. The love of God, squeezed into an arrow, shot forth, and received in the body of a living being, is what brings life to creation. It is inseparable from n|om, and for all practical purposes is n|om, or the most concentrated form of n|om.

The shamans learn to imitate the Sky God, and by feeling a great love, they too tremble and bend over in ecstatic delight. In this transformed state, they are able to both catch and throw an arrow, needle, nail, or thorn. It usually is caught and stored near their belly or near the base of their spine. The shamans also learn to heat the arrow with further shaking. When it gets so hot that the arrow boils and turns to steam, the love and energy (n|om) of the song is released, bringing forth greater ecstatic experience. At this stage, the pump is bringing up the steam from the boiled arrow. It travels up the spine and out through the crown of the head, where it then falls to the ground and cools off, then turns back into an arrow again. Now the Bushman shamans can feel the arrow come through their feet, and the process can be replayed all over again.

The arrows of love, God's thin and sharply pointed holders of love music and rhythm, are boiled, pumped up and out of the body, and then reabsorbed again, over and over. With each recycling, the arrows, needles, and nails are cleaned and revitalized, with the consequence that one's body is also cleaned, revitalized, and recharged. This is how a Bushman maintains health and well-being.

The shamans not only clean and recharge their own arrows, but they also remove other people's arrows and needles, clean them, and reinsert them. Or they simply give people fresh new arrows. The business of a shaman therefore involves catching song arrows, boiling them, and passing them on to others, as well as cleaning and recharging them. The arrows can be caught and sent only through the process of shaking. After a healing dance, the shamans will talk about their arrows and nails, mentioning how they received a new one or how they gave one to someone else. If you haven't heard arrow and needle talk, you haven't spoken shaman's talk with a Bushman.

The release of an arrow is an accurate physical metaphor for what an intensely shaking body sometimes expresses. As you shake, from time to time the intensity builds up to a climactic moment, which is experienced and observed by others as a jolting action. Your body jerks or jolts, feeling and looking as though something is being released. Saying that an arrow has been released fits the phenomenology of what is going on with the body. If a shaman is intensely staring at another person and allowing a buildup of loving emotion toward that person, the subsequent jerk is also understood as the shooting of an arrow into the other person's body. The other person, witnessing this, may then start trembling and shaking. This is a way of sending the shake that does not involve touch, although the other person feels touched.

With the deepest shaking and pumping, the shaman's eyes feel like they are transforming. They call this "getting your second eyes"—seeing with your feelings. In this stage, *synesthesia,* the combining of the senses, becomes more present. Shamans start seeing what they hear (seeing images of the music) and hearing what they see (hearing buzzing sounds that accompany the perception of light). At this time, the perceived world changes. The shamans may feel as though they are floating over the community while seeing various kinds of luminosity. As the shamans become more familiar with this transformation, lines of horizontal light emerge and are recognized as a kind of highway to other places. Shamans find that if they approach one of these lines, they will feel transported to a distant place, perhaps another village or to the location of an animal awaiting the next hunt.

The luminous lines also are seen to extend from the belly of each person to the bellies of everyone else. The white lines are ecstatic realizations of relationships and connections and they are seen through an enhanced state of consciousness brought on by heightened feelings. The shamans learn to see these lines and work with them. The strongest shamans may see the most powerful line, the vertical line or rope that goes straight into the sky. When they walk near this line, they float upward to the sky, entering the great village of the Sky God, who waits to provide teaching. There, they may find ancestors who show them a new dance, sing them a new song, or teach them something, such as pointing out a plant that can be used to heal someone's sickness.

The strongest shamans who travel to the sky village are able to bring the sky down with them when they return. As they float back to Earth, they hold on to the village and bring down all the ancestors. The community below recognizes that this is taking place because its members see the ecstatic emotion on the shaman's face and body. This is the strongest moment in the Bushman healing dance. When the ancestors come down, a moment of eternity is experienced. Here there is no difference among past, present, and future, no sickness, no death. This is when all the loved ones are brought back together through the ceremony of fully opened hearts singing the longings and joys of love.

An old Bushman shaman, |Kunta |Ai!ae, once told me that the rope to God is actually one Bushman ancestor on top of another all the way back to the very first Bushman. When a shaman is training someone, the initiate is sometimes laid over the back of the dancing teacher. A strong shaman is said to be able to "carry many people on his back." The image of stacking one Bushman shaman on the back of another in a line going straight up to the sky was |Kunta's way of explaining the big rope. Experientially, the line connects the Bushman to all ancestors through the link of imagined love. As you love your parents and grandparents, you can further imagine how they loved their parents and grandparents, and on and on until you get to the first ancestors. This line, a love line, is the rope to God.

Over thousands of years, the Bushman shamans have learned how to benefit from shaking medicine. There is more to shaking than trembling and quaking. The shake opens a door to a plethora of experiential outcomes. Shamans use it to express an ecstatic love, to heal, to make emotional contact with their departed love ones, and to transform their experience and relationships with one another. Furthermore, the shaking can be disciplined so it serves to advance the healing and transformation of oneself and others. As the Bushman shaman becomes stronger in the shaking medicine, the door is opened to the most profound ecstatic experiences.

The many different kinds of shaking experience common to Bushman shamans can be used as a reference base for examining other cultures that shake. Shaking medicine can therefore be examined to see whether it includes any or all of the following (with quotations from some of my Bushman teachers over the years—see *Kalahari Bushmen Healers* and *Ropes to God*):

1. Trembling, quaking, shaking, and jerking behavior

   "The spirit touches my feet first during the dance. It then moves through my whole body all the way up to my head. It fills my entire body. It comes up my feet and makes my legs tremble. The trembling shakes the rattles, which are wrapped around my ankles. . . . My belly tightens and vibrates as my entire body starts to shake. Shivering occurs gradually—it builds up to a heavy shaking."

   MABOLELO SHIKWE

   "The spirit makes us shake. . . . The shaking, once it starts, stays with you for the rest of your life. . . . When I shake strongly, it sometimes feels like I have no bones."

   MOTAOPE SABOABUE

   "When I dance, the spirit starts to touch the bottom of my spine. This causes my belly to vibrate. I feel the fire that is responsible for my shaking and vibrating."

   KOMTSA XAU

"When the spirit comes, it enters the base of my spine, and it makes my belly tight and hot. And then I shake. The shaking goes into my entire body."

XIXAE XAU

"In the drum dance, the spirit taps my lower back and then it shoots up my spine to the top of my head. It makes me shake all over."

NXUKA SORIA

2. Inner heat

"It is the power from the music and the seriousness of the occasion that makes me feel very hot. It comes up into my head, and I feel it as a kind of steam that makes my head feel larger."

TWELE

"In the dance, I get hot in my chest. It is painful in the beginning, but then it becomes very nice."

NGWAGA OSELE

"[The power] was so strong that it felt like my arms and body were on fire. The power was hot in my belly and it made me shake."

CGUNTA !ELAE

"This power is like a fire."

TEXAE TOMA

3. Passing on the shake

"The more contact we have between our bodies, the easier it is for me to transfer the [shaking] power. When I place my heart against another person's heart, it helps in transferring my power to them."

MOTAOPE SABOABUE

"When I transfer my spirit to you, I hold you and shake you for a long time. This is a very powerful experience."

KONTSA XAU

"When you transmit the spirit, you hold the other person very tightly. It is like electricity, and it goes right into the other person. Then they start to shake."

XIXAE DXAO

"When you touch someone with this shaking, the power of spirit flows into them. This is the secret of healing. It is the shaking that heals."

MOTAOPE SABOABUE

4. Teaching others how to shake

    "As a teacher of healing, I help others to channel their shaking and body vibrations to grow and mature with their spirits."

    MABOLELO SHIKWE

    "In transferring his spirit, Naledi [the teacher] embraced my whole body and shook me wildly. When he did this, I would also shake."

    RASIMANE

    "When I teach someone to be a doctor, I put power into them."

    CGUNTA !ELAE

5. Shaking inspired by "power" gives way to shaking inspired by "love"

    "Open your heart and serve one another—this is our way. This is the key to healing."

    MABOLELO SHIKWE

    "The secret of the Bushmen is the spirit of joy that we hold in our hearts. Because everyone is part of the whole healing dance, the shivering of the dancers is felt by the people clapping. Any joy that is felt by one person is experienced by everyone."

KAEMME TEBERI

"It's a big day when you first get the big power. . . . The feeling is so intense that you feel your heart breaking and opening to everything in the world."

CGUNTA |KACE

"When I get close to the Big God, I feel his heart. It makes me want to be good to all the people. When I am touching someone with this power, I feel my heart touching my father, my grandfather, and all of their ancestors, all the way to God. . . . That's when I feel everyone's heart."

CGUNTA !ELAE

"When we dance and it's strong, we feel so much emotion that we start crying."

TLIXGO GCAO

6. The shaman's stomping dance and the pump

"With more dancing, the arrows and nails wake up and begin feeling tight in the belly. That makes you bend over and dance in a slower way. That's when you go into the circle toward the fire. . . . You become more ready to doctor the other people."

CGUNTA |KACE

"When you're in the dance and feel your chest and belly get tight, the rope is going through your head and pulling you."

KGAO TEMI

"When I dance, the arrows and nails get heated and my body pumps them up and down."

CGUNTA !ELAE

7. Ecstatic vocalizations

"When I dance and touch someone, I shout loudly."

Ngwaga Osele

"When the power is in you, it can bring out the sounds. There are all kinds of special sounds that can come out of me."

Cgunta !elae

"As the power gets even stronger, it takes over you and it makes noises."

Cgunta |kace

8. Transformational experience (altered visionary, auditory, or olfactory perception and synesthetic experience)

"There are moments in the healing dance when I feel like I am standing in a ray of light. In this light I am able to see inside others."

Mabolelo Shikwe

"I see a light that makes me float. The experience is very wonderful and it feels good."

Twele

"When you see the light in the dance, this means that you are in the world of spirit. You can see sickness and travel to anywhere."

Komtsa Xau

"You see everything at once. Things seem very fast. It all blends together."

Kgao Temi

9. Seeing the "lines" and "ropes"

"When you dance and get hot, you will see a rope hanging from the sky."

Motaope Saboabue

"When you dance, it comes down to you. When it gets into you, you can see it as a string of light."

Xixae Dxao

"When a doctor gets very powerful, he or she will see the rope to God."

Kgao Temi

"The rope is the most important thing we know."

Cgunta |kace

10. Ecstatic imaginary travel

"That line just takes you. The spirit decides where it will take you."

Motaope Saboabue

"The string can take you to another person who needs healing or it can carry you to another village or to the sky."

Xixae Dxao

"Sometimes I travel to another place the instant I go toward a line. At other times you simply walk along it. These lines are all over the land. There are different kinds of lines."

Kgao Temi

11. Learning from the ancestors and gods while in the "spirit world"

"I see my ancestors' faces. They introduce me to my earlier ancestors. . . . They continually teach me about healing and how to live my life."

Mabolelo Shikwe

"My mother brings me magic songs."

Texae Toma

These are some of the experiences the Bushman shakers are familiar with. Some of these outcomes are familiar to other traditions that value and encourage ecstatic expression. What is unique about the Bushmen is the extent to which they have nurtured and developed the shaman's way of shaking to serve the well-being and transformational experiences of their community.

The Bushman shakers teach us that everyone can benefit from the shake. Every week when they hold a healing dance, the shaking shamans touch every member of the community, from infants to elders. Receiving the shake is seen as a medicine both for curing and for maintaining well-being. They use metaphors to describe the shaking medicine that fit the experiences they have with it. Since the entry of a shake into the body may have a tingly or prickly sensation, it is no surprise that they say they have received an arrow or nail. Because they feel an intense heat and sweat profusely during highly aroused shaking, it makes sense that they refer to an internal boiling of their arrows that turns them into steam. When their aroused bodies bring on synesthesia, it isn't surprising that relationships are seen as lines of light and that the music evokes imagined worlds with longed-for ancestors.

In the Kalahari and in other places of the world, I have shaken myself into the mysteries. I have seen and journeyed along the lines and climbed the rope to God. I have shaken myself into the light and into the transformations that still the mind and body. My entry was facilitated by giving no inappropriate importance to the abstracted lines and partial approximations produced by the traditions of discourse and text. I used them, but was not attached to them. The Bushmen taught me to let the metaphors and meanings slip and slide, change, shape-shift, transform, and evaporate. Shaking the words and the meanings is as important as shaking the bodies. The two are inseparable.

After the shaking takes place, the Bushmen taught me another use of words. They use words to keep themselves free from getting stuck to any over-importance attributed to their shaking experiences and visionary experiences. If you shake all night and travel to the sky, there is a temptation to say the next morning, "I found the truth." Then you get stuck and start to evangelize a truth that others need to recognize and accept. As sociologists of religion discuss this process, charismatic (ecstatic) experiences are typically "routinized" into rituals of performance and social institutions. The consequence of institutionalization is that the originating inspiration and experience often go away. This constitutes the routinization of the spirit.

The Bushmen protect themselves from routinization by not allowing anyone to take their experiential outcomes too seriously. The morning after a dance, talk is used to tease and make fun of one another in a kind and friendly manner. Even though they recognize that there are natural hierarchies of ability and performance in the community, they do not allow anyone to get carried away by it. For instance, if a man returns with a lot of meat after a successful hunt, the community will tease him, even suggesting that he had sex with the animal in order to get it to give up its life for him.

Similarly, the Bushmen celebrate the ecstatic truths of their dance by laughing and teasing one another when it is over. This keeps them unattached to any form, permitting transformation to blow through again. They honor the shifting of the forms, not any particular form. This Earth-grounded wisdom is not far removed from Buddhism, with its teachings of being unattached so that people may move more gracefully with the truth of never-ceasing change. Similarly, the Christian counsel to lose one's life in order to find it requires being moved by and constantly moving with the Holy Spirit.

The Bushmen's shaking medicine and the metaphors used to describe the experiences associated with it enable us to deepen our understanding of how heightened arousal can contribute to our lives. Shaking can be approached in two different ways. You can start with the behavior of shaking and hope that it leads you into the bigger experiences, ultimately culminating with a mystical realization of ecstatic love, or you can start with an inspired love and allow its heart-opening power to bring forth the shaking and quaking.

As we saw in the previous chapter, Western scholars and researchers start with a simple action and use it to open doors to higher consciousness. Cultural wisdom traditions, however, start from the top, with the love and honoring of the great mysteries, ancestors, spirits, celestial beings, and gods, and allow that experience to trickle down, bringing forth trembling. Remember that the Western methods that start from simple actions typically have to keep adding more contextual pieces in order to enhance their effects. This finding suggests that the more you move toward mystery and communicate an openness to the divine, independent of whether or not you understand it, the more enhanced are the arousal, the love, and the transformational outcomes.

The Bushmen free themselves from having to decide whether they will start with the particular action and then build up the context or they will aim for the top and let it spill forth the ecstatic blessings. They see the line as a circle in which it doesn't matter whether you think you are at the top or at the bottom, because it is all connected. When you shake, you are aware of the great mysteries, and when you consider the great love and presence of the gods, you shake. Climbing the rope to God and coming down with the sky village is turning the line into a circle. What momentarily looks like a straight line is, from a different perspective, only a fragment of a larger arc. As a simple example, we look at a tennis court and see that the court's portion of the earth is flat, but we also know that it is part of an arc of land that is inseparable from the curvature of the spherical Earth.

A line that is cut from the larger arcs and circles that hold it can potentially breed trouble and suffering. In other words, the problem with reductionism isn't its act of reduction, but rather forgetting that it first cut out a piece from a greater whole. Acting as if the part of the line is the whole sets up all kinds of fallacious assumptions that easily precipitate contextual dis-ease. When an abstracted part or line is seen as separate from the whole, it tempts us to think in terms of maximizing and minimizing certain aspects, qualities, and characteristics. For example, the maximization of resources on the planet without considering how they affect the whole ecosystem is an error of this kind. This applies to the non-tempered accumulation of wealth, petroleum, and lumber, among other resources.

Systemic wisdom never forgets that all the parts are inseparable from their whole context. It enables us to see that lines are parts of bigger circles and that our love for our family is part of a bigger love for community and planet, all the way to an infinite, unknowable mystery. The Bushman shamans suggest that as we honor and enact relationships with the greater contexts and circles of life, our minds surpass and exhaust their ability to rationally comprehend the increased complexity and connectivity. As we pass the limits of mind, it becomes easier to expand our capacity for expression. The stilled mind frees an ecstatic body. If you want to stop thinking, then start shaking. You can't think in the midst of ecstatic body fervor.

With an empty mind, we are able to fully surrender to a body that wants to perform, to shake itself into ecstatic delight. The body, in turn, eventually reaches its natural limit and collapses to an even greater stillness and quietude. Here, both mind and body hand themselves over to the deepest silences and mysteries of soul. When soul comes forth, we find ourselves inseparable from one another and from the greater wholes that hold us. Unknowable, impossible to express, the great void, the whole universe affirms its mystery and presence. Here, with the mystics, we become whole and holy.

The shaking medicine of the Bushmen is a worship of transformation, the wind of change, what the Dine call Nilch'i. Akin to the Holy Spirit, it suffuses all of nature and brings forth life, thought, speech, and motion. It enters and leaves us through the whorls of our fingers and toes and the whorl on the top of our head. As with n|om, we must learn to be moved by it and move with it. This movement is exalted when we spiritually tremble, quake, and shake. In this sacred movement, we are tuned and brought back into the natural order, made more present in the Taoist's *wu-wei*, the natural wisdom that determines when to act and when not to act.

The Bushman shakers teach us to move past the fear of being out of control and turn ourselves over to another process of control that shakes our bodies. As we become comfortable in the shake, we see that it carries us deeper into other opportunities of surrender. We can sacrifice the sense of power that shaking first suggests, and humbly allow love rather than power to govern the movements.

In the movement to heart, our deepest longings pull us toward the lines and ropes of relationship. In the center of relationship, we lose our self again and find our self-centered mind to be empty of content. We move into the mind and heart of relationship. Here the ecstatic heat continues to intensify and come to a boil. As thoughts melt and give way to rhythms and music, the heaviness of physical and mental gravity is reduced to steam and wind. As we ascend and descend the spiritual ropes, holding on to the transforming arrows of love, our identity gives way to a greater presence of soul. Here, there is only light and movement and the realization of an unspeakable mystery that unifies all creation. Here we enter the mind and heart of God.

All Bushman shamans go through several stages of mastery, beginning with learning to be comfortable with shaking. In the beginning stage, the trembling, quaking, and shaking bring forth a sense of power. Shamans learn to heat up and shake. At this stage, because of the emphasis upon personal power, shamans are more likely to define their shamanic role as fighting off malevolent spirits.

The next stage of development for the Bushman shamans takes place when the inspiration for their shaking begins shifting from power to love. As they learn to move the shaking energy into their heart, they feel compassion toward the sick. Then their trembling hands touch others, trying to remove the sickness. Here the pump is emphasized, along with the vocalizations it produces. Now there is more singular focus, and shamans may start seeing (through feelings) the luminous lines and have experiences of traveling along them.

In the most advanced stage, Bushman shamans move fully to love-inspired shaking. They feel a love not only for their living relatives and departed ancestors, but also for the Sky God and all of creation. They even feel a love for their enemies. This is the highest level of transformation. The strongest shamans see and feel the ropes to God and they go up them. They are the doctor's doctors, the shaman's shamans. They revitalize the other shamans. In this highest state, shamans may feel the loss of physical form and perceive a transformation into a vibrating cloud of energy. As Motaope Saboabue once told me: "You may even forget that you have a body and think that you are a mist or a cloud. This is the way it must be. This proves you are a powerful medicine man."

We can use these stages of development—beginning, middle, and advanced shaking—to examine any shaker's development and form of expression. We can apply it to particular individuals as well as to cultures that practice shaking. As we turn to other cultures, we will see that they each teach us something about shaking medicine. We will compare their practice to what we have learned from the world's oldest culture, that of the Bushman shakers, and aim to expand our understanding of the nature and practice of shaking.

Before proceeding, I want to tell a story about one of the times I was traveling to southern Africa to visit my Bushman friends. While sitting on a South African Airlines flight, the person sitting next to me introduced himself as a South African physician. When he found out I had been visiting the Bushmen, he became very excited and said he had been the physician for the film crew during the making of the movie *The Gods Must Be Crazy*. Later in our conversation, he said that something had happened during that time that puzzled him to this day.

The doctor mentioned that during the filming, the star of the film, a Bushman named N!xau, became very ill and went off to recover. When they found him, he was sitting under a tree in a trance as his body shook wildly. No one could tell what was wrong, and as they drove him to reach a hospital, he continued to shake. Before they came to the hospital, over a full day's drive away, N!xau stopped shaking and started talking as if nothing was wrong. He had fully recovered. "To this day I don't know what happened to the Bushman," the doctor told me. I tried to explain that shaking was the way the Bushmen often heal themselves. The doctor had witnessed the oldest and newest cure on Earth.

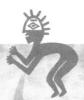

4

THE LAST TABOO

Why Did the Quakers Stop Quaking and the Shakers Stop Shaking?

Why did the Quakers stop quaking and the Shakers stop shaking? Is it related to why the majority of technologically developed cultures all but eliminated shaking bodies from public performance, worship, and healing encounters? I will argue that ecstatic shaking is the last great taboo for the technologically developed (but spiritually underdeveloped) world. Studying what happened to the shake and quake in Europe and North America will show that the greatest fear about the body does not necessarily concern sexual expression, but instead liberation of the body into full-flight ecstatic expression.

Seeing shaking, quaking, and sometimes convulsing bodies calls forth the social labels of "madness," "neurological disorder," "psychological dissociation," and "possession by evil spirits." Most of us, along with the quieted Shakers and Quakers, have stopped shaking because what we fear most is being out of control or being seen by others as sick, bad, or mad. Yet the paradox of human experience is that we seek the transcendent experience that requires us to surrender control. A historical examination of what happened to the Quakers and Shakers may help us understand how to overcome this fear and taboo, opening the door for the shaking medicine to return in a good way.

There was tremendous religious and political upheaval in England during the middle of the seventeenth century. It was a time of horrible imprisonment, irrational cruelty, and great social tension. In that time of suffering, people, particularly those among the poor, began proclaiming miracles, prophecies, and shaking ecstasy. One of the main spiritual figures to arise was George Fox, credited with the formation of the Quaker religion. Born in Drayton-in-the-Clay, Leicestershire, Fox learned to be a shoemaker. As a young man, he desperately wanted to directly experience God, rather than merely be faithful to the teachings of spiritual authorities. After receiving a small inheritance, he began traveling, hoping to find a way to satisfy his spiritual hunger. He met many "ranters," preachers who believed they communed with God but belonged to no church. In spite of those encounters, he remained unsatisfied and decided to return home. On his way back, in 1647, he had a spiritual revelation that he described in his diary:

> But as I had forsaken the priests, so I left the separate preachers also . . . for I saw there was none among them all that could speak to my condition. And when all my hopes in them and in all men were gone, so that I had nothing outwardly to help me, nor could tell what to do, then, Oh, then, I heard a voice which said, "There is one, even Christ Jesus, that can speak to thy condition," and when I heard it, my heart did leap for joy.[1]

What was radical about Fox was that he brought forth his spiritual experience by experimenting with the divine. He set aside religious teachings, including the Bible, and faithfully waited for God to speak. Once he made experiential contact with the divine, he did not want to stop its transmission of ecstatic revelation:

> My desires for the Lord grew stronger, and zeal in the pure knowledge of God, and Christ alone, without the help of any man, book, or writing. For though I read the Scriptures that spoke of Christ and of God, yet I knew Him not, but by revelation. . . . The Lord did gently lead me along, and did let me see His love, which was end-

less and eternal, surpasseth all the knowledge that men have in the natural state, or can obtain from history or books.[2]

Fox, a large man with piercing eyes, dressed in a leather suit, went about the country by foot and slept under the trees. He believed that "a great work of the Lord fell on me," and thought he could read the character of people by looking at them. He healed people with the touch of his hands, and his preaching brought forth shaking and quaking in the congregation. Often beaten, stoned, and run out of town, he was sent to prison eight times. He was best known for the power of his praying. He would begin in silence, waiting for the spirit to come upon him. Then when he began to speak with an inspired voice, the whole congregation would start shaking: "As the power of God came down in such a marvelous manner the very building seemed to rock."[3]

George Fox soon claimed to have the gifts of clairvoyance, prophecy, and healing. Once, while walking barefoot through the town of Lichfield, he envisioned a river of blood flowing through its streets. He shouted, "Woe to the bloody city of Lichfield!" He later discovered that Christians had been murdered there some thirteen centuries before. At another time, while in the streets of London, he spent two days proclaiming that a great fire was coming. In 1666, the great fire of London did occur, further establishing Fox's prophetic talent.

Fox developed his gifts through frequent fasting and long walks in solitary places. He would sit in a hollow tree with his Bible or take long walks by himself at night. Once, he fell into a trance that lasted some fourteen days. When he awakened, his personal suffering was lifted, and "with brokenness of heart and tears of joy, he acknowledged the infinite love of God."[4]

Originally called the Children of the Light, Fox's followers were later called Quakers because of the violent trembling that came upon them when they worshipped. As people experienced the "inner light of the spirit," they realized and professed that all human beings, rich and poor, educated and uneducated, were equal. Furthermore, they asserted that the true Christian had an "indwelling life of Christ" that was more important than the scriptures. It was the inner spirit that could reveal the truth of the Bible, not a socially anointed religious authority. They rejected worldly values and sought "religious perfection." Wild shaking and convulsing, unexpected behavior, unique visions, curing the sick, working miracles, long fasts, and even a form of holy nudism were explored. The early Quakers would give voice to wild sounds when under the influence of the spirit:

> The Devil roared in these deceived souls [one witness recalls] in a most strange and dreadful Manner, some howling, some shrieking, yelling, roaring, and some had a strange confused kind of humming, singing Noise . . . about the one Half of these miserable Creatures were terribly shaken with violent Motions.[5]

The Quakers rejected liturgical structure, administration, and ordination, and preferred being obedient only to the spirit. When they gathered for a meeting, they waited in silence until the spirit announced itself, and then anything could happen. This religious practice did not sit well with the secular and religious authorities.

Judith Rose writes that "Fox's assertion that true knowledge comes directly from God without the intercession of writing—or even of speech itself—challenges the whole rhetorical structure upon which seventeenth century thought is built."[6] Those who based their faith on written or spoken words rather than direct divine experience were called "thieves" by some of the Quakers. Like shamans of old and the still-practicing Bushman shaking shamans, Fox and the Quakers valued ecstatic experience as the primary source of wisdom and expression.

The Quakers explored the kingdom within. They saw heaven, hell, and the resurrection as stages of internal development. By rejecting social authority, instead turning to the authority of ecstatic experience, they were explorers of the spiritual wilderness. They encouraged and allowed any statements to be made and any actions to be performed as long as there was divine inspiration. Following George Fox, they practiced experimental spirituality.

Individual and social outbursts of ecstatic expression and shaking were historically known in Europe and other parts of the world. Enthusiastic dancing was part of the ancient Hebrew tradition, and even King David "danced before the Lord with all his might" (2 Samuel 6:14). Muhammad had convulsions during which he received the visions and revelations that led to a whole religion. It is uncertain as to whether he had epilepsy or hysteria or was simply in spiritual ecstasy. He even doubted his own sanity for a while.

In the 1300s, so-called epidemics of wild religious dancing broke out in Europe, from the lower Rhine to the Netherlands and France. Hundreds, if not thousands, started dancing in the streets, in churches, and in their homes, claiming to honor St. John. They would dance for hours and hours until they fell to the ground in shaking fits of ecstasy. They too shouted wild cries and had visions. The dance was contagious, and the religious and political authorities demanded that exorcism be used to stop the disease. In the 1400s, the wild dancing broke out again, this time called St. Vitus' dance. The trembling bodies were again diagnosed by the clergy and sent to the church of St. Vitus at Rotestein for healing prayers to calm them down.

As we approach the age of the Quakers and Shakers, there were also ecstatics called the French Prophets. They attracted a lot of attention because their shaking was vigorously enthusiastic, described as being "violent agitations of the body."[7] Men, women, and children were part of this movement. They all shook and had visions. Once, Charles Wesley spent the night with a member of this religious group. Charles, along with his brother John Wesley, was one of the founders of Methodism and is remembered today for the many hymns he wrote, including "Hark! The Herald Angels Sing" and "O for a Thousand Tongues to Sing." One night, as Charles was about to go to bed, his friend fell into an ecstatic state, shook wildly, and started gobbling like a turkey. Wesley thought he was possessed by the devil, so he started exorcising him. Later, he visited a prophetess of the group to see where the spirits came from. She began shaking and convulsing and then spoke with a clear authoritative voice, leading her observers to believe that she was speaking for God.

There were also the Jumpers, known for singing a song over and over as a means to bring on ecstatic experience. After singing a song thirty to forty times with all their might, people would start shaking and jumping up and down for hours. In this social climate, it should not be surprising that when John Wesley started preaching, people also started to shake, an outcome he regarded as a "great triumph." John Wesley describes the experiences that took place at one of his services:

> While I was earnestly inviting all men to enter into the Holiest by this new and living way, many of those that heard began to call upon God with strong cries and tears. Some sank down, and there remained no strength in them. Others exceedingly trembled and quaked. Some were torn with a kind of convulsive motion in every part of their bodies, and that so violently that often four or five persons could not hold one of them. I have seen many hysterical and epileptic fits, but none of them were like these in many respects.[8]

There was a lot of shaking going on in England during the 1700s, and it never failed to upset the religious and secular authorities. Not surprisingly, George Fox was sent to prison in 1649 for violating the blasphemy law. He continued to denounce both religious authorities and civil legal authorities, challenging the entire structure of society. Another prominent Quaker and ranter, James Nayler, was also arrested, for riding into town on an ass surrounded by a group of women. Hoping to find a safe place to practice their faith, boatloads of shakers fled to North America. Tired of persecution, in 1657 some Quakers boarded the ship *The Woodhouse* and sailed for the American colonies.

George Fox was one of them. One of the more interesting consequences of the spirited free expression associated with Fox's Quakerism was that he permitted women to have an equal voice. As he declared, "Christ in the Male, and in the Female is one." Nearly half the Quakers who went to America were women who were filled with heightened fervor and had no fear about expressing themselves. When touched by the spirit, they were as bold as the Old Testament prophets.

Fox stopped in Barbados to convert a small number of colonists and then went on to convert the settlers and Indians of Maryland, New Jersey, and New England. His friend William Penn described him as "an original, being no man's copy." It didn't take long for the ecstatic Quakers, or Friends, as they called themselves, to be called witches and heretics. A tract distributed in 1653 entitled *Brief Relation of the Irreligion of the Northern Quakers* proposes: "I heartily believe these quakings to be diabolical raptures." Robert Barclay, in another tract, wrote: "The Friends . . . occasionally administered a cordial or medicine of some kind, and this is commented upon in the tracts of the times as a circumstance of the utmost mystery and a proof of sorcery!"[9]

It didn't matter that the Quakers quoted the Bible to defend their quaking, pointing out that Moses "quaked," David "roared," and Jeremiah "trembled." They were still found guilty of harboring evil ways. Some were dunked, bridled, whipped, bored through the tongue with a hot iron, branded on the forehead with the letter *B* (for *blasphemer*), and sent to jail. As persecution continued over the years, the Quakers gave up their ecstatic and prophetic role in society and changed to being calm advocates of education and organized meetings. The quaking stopped along with their persecution. The taboo against quaking and shaking had been maintained.

While in England, it had taken George Fox only ten years to convert some sixty thousand men and women to his charismatic faith. Today, there are fewer than seventeen thousand Quakers in all of Great Britain. And all Quakers throughout the world have essentially stopped quaking. Quaker and syndicated columnist David Yount wrote an essay in 2002 asking the question "Why Did Quakers Stop Quaking?" He was responding to a personal challenge from a Pentecostal minister who suggested that the Quakers had lost their originating fervor. Yount replied, "I believe the response that popped into my head that day was pretty good. I suggested to him that Quakers stopped quaking when we stopped being persecuted."

I suggest that the opposite is true: the Quakers stopped quaking because they were persecuted, even imprisoned, for their wild ecstatic experiences. When they were obedient to the truth of ecstatic expression, they were unable to stop quaking. Yount ended his essay by providing another answer, more in tune with this latter perspective. He quotes an elder Quaker in his eighties who gave this response: "I know why I don't quake. I don't ask God the hard questions about what he requires me to do with my life. I'm afraid that if I ask him, God will tell me something difficult that I'm unwilling to do. But if I was willing to listen to him, and do what he demands, then I'd start quaking."

When the Quakers were persecuted by the colonial Puritans, some moved to the American wilderness and lived with the Indians.[10] There they found a mutual understanding and respect of personal revelation and spiritual experience. The Indians and Quakers got along quite well. The same goodwill toward the Indians was also found with the early Shakers.

The Shakers were arguably an offshoot of the Quakers. Started by Ann Lee, they came from Manchester, England, to America in 1774, also seeking a place to worship free from persecution. Shakerism subsequently became an American movement located mostly in New England and New York. Ann Lee was the daughter of a blacksmith. Like George Fox, she had looked for a more personal relationship with the divine. Her marriage had been miserable, and after her four children died in birth or infancy, she began having visions. Soon after, she was believed to have the "Christ spirit" within her and was called Mother Ann, a "Mother in spiritual things."

When it came to matters of spirit, Mother Ann didn't hold back. She was frequently imprisoned for dancing and shouting on the Sabbath. Her followers were called Shakers because of their rituals of trembling, shouting, singing, speaking in tongues, and especially shaking their bodies. They became so ecstatic that they sometimes rolled on the floor or jumped and danced while having visions and trances.

Like the Quakers, the Shakers believed in personal communication with a God who was both male and female. They became famous for their swaying movements and dances brought about by the spirit. Their intense ecstatic worship led to dramatic spiritual manifestations. For example, children and adults claimed to visit cities in the spiritual realm and deliver messages from angels. One of their members, Frederick W. Evans, provides a personal account of their ecstatic experience:

> Sometimes, after sitting awhile in silent meditation, they were seized with a mighty trembling, under which they would often express the indignation of God against all sin. At other times they were exercised with singing, shouting, and leaping for joy at the near prospect of salvation. They were often exercised with great agitation of body and limbs, shaking, running, and walking the floor, with a variety of other operations and signs, swiftly passing and repassing each other like clouds agitated with a mighty wind. These exercises, so strange in the eyes of the beholders, brought upon them the appellation of Shakers, which has been their name of distinction ever since. . . . And whatever manner the spirit may dictate, or whatever the form into which the spirit may lead, it is acceptable to Him from whom the spirit proceeds . . . (on one particular occasion) previous to our coming we called a meeting and there was so many gifts (such as prophecies, revelations, visions, and dreams) in confirmation of a former revelation for us to come that some could hardly wait for others to tell their gifts. We had a joyful meeting and danced till morning.[11]

Not surprisingly, given her experience with marriage and childbearing, Mother Ann called for the advocacy of celibacy. She fought against "wallowing in the lusts" and denied herself the pleasures of sexuality, sleep, food, and drink. She became so weak that she sometimes had to be fed by others. In her services, the men and women were separated so they wouldn't touch each other during their shaking fits. Elders would make sure that no touching occurred between the sexes.

Mother Ann went on a mission to spread her truth and covered most of southern New England. The native people of New England felt a kindred connection with her. One Indian, after meeting Mother Ann, said he had seen a bright light around her and was convinced she had been sent by the Great Spirit. When Mother Ann and her followers arrived in New York, they chose to live in an isolated wilderness area, a swampland called Niskayuna (now Watervliet). It didn't take long for persecution to begin. Among other things, they were charged for inciting the Indians against the government.

Mother Ann died on September 8, 1784, but her spiritual impact continued. Over half a century later, during February 1837, a spiritual revival began sweeping through the Shaker communities; it was called "Mother's Work." Often occurring in children, it would begin with involuntary jerks and shaking movements that would lead to a trance. The practitioner would then claim to have contact with Indian spirits. Some even began speaking in the Indian language. The Indian spirits were visioned along with the spirits of Jesus and Mother Ann. Spiritual gifts received during this time of trances, spinning, and wild shaking included visions, revelations, prophecies, and songs.

One specialized service was called a "quick meeting" or "Shaker high." It would begin with an elder commenting that all good believers were known by the variety of their gifts. He would then shout, "Shake off the flesh!" and immediately start stomping and shaking. Haskett describes what would then take place:

> In an instant the spirit seized all the members; and one continued shout, and tremendous noise of stamping was only to be heard. . . (then the whole room would) shake, jump, and turn. . . . Then commenced an awful riot. Now was heard the loud shouts of the brethren, then the soft, but hurried notes of the sisters, whose "gifts" were the apostolic gifts of the tongues. These gently gestured their language, waved themselves backward and forward like a ship on the billows of a ceased storm, shook their heads, seized their garments, and then violently stamped on the floor.[12]

During this time of spiritual revival, Elder William Reynolds, of Union Village, Ohio, at the age of sixty-five, started the ecstatic practice of turning cartwheels from his home to church, sometimes turning over fences. He did this every Sunday for three years.[13] There were also well-documented reports of clairvoyant communication among different church groups. It was a time of fervent shaking, visionary experience, and altered states of consciousness. Even the Indian ways entered into their rituals. Some Shakers smoked an Indian medicine pipe, participated in purification rites similar to the sweat lodge, bathed in spiritual waters, and readily received guidance from Indian spirits.

It wasn't only the Shakers who were shaking, having visions, and shamanizing in early American history. Among the Free Will Baptists of New England, "Tumult reigned and 'strong men fell as if slain in battle.'"[14] The Primitive Baptists of Virginia would "roar on the ground, ring their hands, go into ecstasies, pray and weep while others did so much outrageous cursing and swearing that it was thought they were really possessed of the devil."[15]

In 1805, several Shakers heard about trembling and spasmodic movements taking place in the revivals of Kentucky. Thinking this was similar to their own shaking, they took off on a journey to see what was taking place, hoping it would be an opportunity to spread the Shaker religion.

Shaker missionaries did expand their religion into the area. In spite of their competitive rivalry, the Shakers and Kentucky revivalists influenced one another, each borrowing and modifying ritualistic aspects from the other. It wasn't long before the Shakers used Baptist and Methodist hymns and the various groups of the Kentucky revival started dancing. During this time, various observers noticed the "rolling exercise," the "jerks," and the "barks," all of which became familiar to the Shakers. Blinn writes:

One of the most singular manifestations was that of the "jerks." These were not particularly interesting or instructive, and many times they must have been very distasteful to the actor. The head would be twitched from side to side and at times with extreme velocity. The arms would be thrown involuntarily in every direction, and this would often take place in the dining hall, and even when engaged in manual occupation in the shop or in the field. Sometimes it would occur while the medium was on the highway, very much to his own mortification, and quite as much so, perhaps to his friends. With his arms spasmodically thrown out and violently jerked back, he certainly must have presented a very singular appearance and have been subjected to the derision of the general observer.[16]

The jerks, jumps, and hops were sometimes expressed with the "barks." Writing about the Kentucky revivalists, McNemar observed that a person would assume "the position of a canine beast, move about on all fours, growl, snap the teeth, and bark," sometimes at the foot of a tree in what was called "treeing the devil." People would disengage from the grip of this activity by moving into vigorous dancing.

In the early spring of 1838, the Shakers' spiritual ecstasies reached a new level. The Shaker historian Isaac Youngs wrote that "the windows of heaven and the avenues of the spirit world set open." For over a decade, Shaker visionaries appeared to be possessed by and to speak, sing, or act in the name of various spirits. It was common for inspired people or "instruments" to start shaking and convulsing or wildly whirling until they fell to the ground, looking as if they had died. They might stay in that trance state for hours or days. When they were lifted up, they would speak in a clear voice, bringing spiritual messages to the community.

I earlier referred to this as the time of Mother's Work. The initial transmission came from Mother Ann and Jesus, followed by other spirits with names like the Angel of Love, Gabriel, Sounding Angel, and the Angel of Consuming Fire, as well as Samuel, Elijah, Ezekiel, Daniel, Napoleon, Washington, Alexander the Great—and William Penn. Sometimes they brought spiritual gifts—that is, announcements of special items that would have spiritual importance or power for particular individuals. These spiritual gifts included fruits and flowers; diamonds, emeralds, sapphires, and other precious stones; golden bowls and chains; boxes filled with treasures; cakes of love, silver cups filled with the pure love of Christ and Mother, plates of wisdom, baskets of simplicity, balls of promise, belts of wisdom, bands of brightness, and robes of meekness; heavenly doves; leaves from the tree of life; rods of correction or comfort; sharp swords, breastplates of truth, and shining armor; cards of love, sacred sheets, drawings, paintings, and other symbolic designs; peace pipes, flags, trumpets, and spiritual wine.[17] When a person was told about the gift, he or she would pantomime receiving and using it. The gift of spiritual wine "carried a great evidence of its reality, by the paroxysms of intoxication which it produced, causing those who drank it to stagger and reel, like drunken people."[18]

Some Shakers even received the "laughing gift," and "laughing songs" in which they held their sides, laughing themselves into exhaustion. Musical instruments were delivered to them as well as specialized rhythms and songs. One song, called "The Sound," involved the rhythmic beating of their hands against the floor. As usual, the reception of spiritual gifts and revelations was accompanied by wild shaking.

An account of receiving a spiritual gift is given in David Lamson's *Two Years' Experience Among the Shakers:*

Holy Mother: Elder William, do you consider this brother a good Believer?

Elder William: Yea, I consider that brother David has good faith, understanding faith; and is endeavoring to live up to it.

Holy Mother: Yea, truly it must be so.

David (repeating after an Elder Sister): Holy Holy Mother Wisdom! I thank thee for thy great condescension and blessing, and for thy love and mercy to me.

Holy Mother (kneeling): Around thy head I place a golden band. On it is written the name of me, Holy Mother wisdom! The Great Jehovah! The Eternal God! Touch not mine anointed.

As the medium spoke, she went through the motions of placing a band on the person's head. After the gift was received, the person bowed seven times with gratitude.

Some of the most welcomed spiritual gifts were the songs people received while in an ecstatic state. Poole writes:

> Witness the sweet . . . melodies which come (from) "the gift of the spirit," as they believe, to one or another, either in private or in public worship. A brother or sister at such times is inspired to sing a new song to new music, which, when written down, becomes a permanent possession. A large book has been published, consisting of these inspirational hymns, which is in constant use.[19]

The height of the Shaker practice of receiving spiritual gifts took place in 1842, when many of their most elaborate rituals were conceived, including the "Midnight Cry" (marching through the room of every building), the "Sweeping Gift" (cleaning houses, shops, and premises with spiritual brooms), "Winding March," "Lively Line," "Changeable Dance," "Cross and Diamond," "Lively Ring," "Square and Compass," various mountain meetings, "taking in the spirits of Indians," the sowing of "spiritual seeds," and bathing in spiritual waters.

During that same year, local hills and mountains, among other places, were renamed with holy names such as Mt. Sinai (at Hancock, Massachusetts), Holy Hill of Zion (at Harvard, Massachusetts), Holy Mount (at Enfield, Connecticut). For the next three years, Shaker services were closed to the public as the Shakers began taking semiannual pilgrimages to their newly named sacred sites. They would fast and pray before dressing in imaginary clothing, received from an imaginary chest. The clothing included a coat of twelve colors, white slacks, and a silver fur hat for the men and a gown of twelve colors, silver-colored shoes and bonnets, and blue silk gloves for the women. As Lamson explains:

> On this day, the brethren and sisters wear their usual Sunday clothes, and in addition a most splendid Spiritual dress. This dress cannot be seen by the natural eye, but is described by the Seers, who can see Spiritual things. . . . Every society has its chest of this

spiritual clothing. . . . Some of the inspired ones at Enfield, saw the angels bring this box, or chest, into the room. . . . And so we are clothed. . . . It is said that in one instance, one of the Seers, in folding, and laying this clothing into the chest, counted the garments, and one suit was missing. The fact was, one of the sisters failed to return hers with the rest, being engaged at the time about some domestic affairs. Now does this not prove the thing to be a reality?[20]

After being dressed up for the pilgrimage, the Shakers would then sing and march up a holy hill as imaginary incense was poured over them. With the announcement that it was time for a "lively dance," the brethren were invited to "strip off their coats" and "go to work." They would then leap into a frenzy of ecstatic expression, skipping, rolling on the ground, shouting, bowing, clapping, and whirling, all as an acknowledgment of "the mighty power of the Lord." Lamson provides this first-person account:

Joseph Wicker . . . comes forth from the rest, and is within the ring: bowing and twisting his body in various directions, his eyes and lips in rapid motion. . . . This is to signify that he is under the influence of inspiration. Or, as they term it, he is "under operations" . . . [m]any declare, "The Lord is here.". . . And a general excitement seems to pervade the meeting. Various are the operations with which those are seized who are easily wrought upon. Twisting, jerking, bowing, trembling, etc. One sister now appears within the ring turning round as rapidly as the roughness of the ground will allow her to . . . she is taken with a mighty bowing; bringing her face oftentimes nearly to the ground; and motioning with her right hand in a very strange and mysterious manner.

Once the spirited expression was set loose, people would soon speak and sing in tongues as spiritual gifts were dispersed. Spiritual wine would be drunk from imaginary bottles, followed by the singing of a "fool-song," sung while everyone acted foolish so as to vex any self-conceit:

> *Come, come, who will be a fool,*
> *I will be a fool—*

Other rituals followed, including the firing of spiritual guns at invisible enemies and the sprinkling of holy love over all the faithful. Eventually, "small papers of seed" were placed in "spiritual baskets" to be sowed over the holy ground. Watered by holy water, it was believed that they would bring forth great blessings.

When this was completed, the elders would sometimes invite the Indian spirits to join their dance. The people would begin to whoop, hop on one foot, dance sideways, and run back and forth, believing they were giving and receiving love. Other cultural spirits entered them, including African tribes, Peruvians, Patagonians, Laplanders, Siberians, Arabs, Irish, Scotts, French, Spanish, Grecians, Persians, Turks, Moors, Chinese, Jews, and Abyssinians. At one mountain meeting, the Shakers estimated they were visited by forty thousand spirits! Blinn describes the multicultural display:

> Under the influence of the Indian spirits they would shout and dance and then give their war whoop. Some acted precisely the peculiar traits of the Negro, Arab, the Chinese, or even the politeness of the French. They conversed, and each class seemed to understand their own company, but to the spectators it was peculiarly amusing.[21]

At the end of these possessions and rituals, the community celebrated with a spiritual feast that served even more spiritual wine. The food, consisting of fruit, turkey, chicken, pudding, pies, green corn, and beans, was all imaginary, though "the inspired ones pretended they could positively see, and taste the different articles of fruit, and food, as if they were literally food."[22] When they went home, they were so filled with spiritual food that there was no hunger for natural food.

For the purest of hearts, the love of God brought them into experiences of rapture, as was the case with James Whitaker, described and quoted by F. W. Evans:

> With tears rolling down his eyes, he frequently expressed his love to God, and his thankfulness for the Gospel, in the following language: "O how precious is the way of God to my thirsty soul! I feel the love of God continually flowing into my soul, like rivers of living water! It is sweeter to my taste than honey in the honey-comb! I know that God owns me for his son, and yet I will pray to Him. I know how to pray, and I know how to be thankful for the Gospel. Even my breath is continual prayer to God."[23]

The Shakers were well aware that their spiritual performances looked "silly to the natural mind." It took spiritual eyes to see that what took place was the work of angels and spirits. One had to be in the spirit, and often not conscious, to allow spirit to act through one's body. The proof of spiritual presence was in the frenzied behavior.

Upon occasion, someone would take on a spirit that would manifest "wicked" behavior. For example, one young man would start cursing and ridiculing the religious life. He was cured when another possessed person, supposedly using the voice of Mother Ann, gave him a scolding. He immediately asked for forgiveness: "Pardon! Pardon! O forgive my transgressions!"[24]

The Shakers understood that different kinds of gifts were brought through the spirit and that some were more desirable than others. They believed that "the character of these spirits is in some degree determined by the character and willed purpose of the earthly inhabitant . . . the lesson is that kindred spirits attract each other . . . to the pure in heart and life the ministrations from the spirit world will emanate from the sainted throng who dwell in the mansions of God's truth and love; and the inspirations from these are heaven born and true."[25] The Shakers found that the form and quality of spirited expression depended on the form and quality of the human performer. An "unclean instrument" could easily channel stupidity or irrational anger, whereas a "clean, inspired instrument" could voice great beauty and wisdom. The quality of a person's unconscious expression was often the same quality as his or her conscious offerings. An ignorant man or woman was typically just as unenlightened under the influence of spirit. A spiritual life served to prepare both one's conscious and unconscious mind to be a purveyor of wisdom. This helps explain why the Shakers were so determined to live an ascetic life. They wanted to be worthy vehicles who would attract the highest spirits to come through them.

In 1848, the Fox sisters of Hydesville, New York (no relation to George Fox), started the spiritualism movement. Some scholars have proposed that the Shakers were their inspiration, but, in fact, when the Shakers invited mediums to perform in their services, the Shakers were offended. The lack of religious ecstasy showed that the spiritualists weren't spiritually inspired. Youngs wrote in 1850 that "to us it has afforded but little benefit; and we are satisfied that this form of communion with the spirit world is not for Believers in our faith."[26] To the Shakers, shaking inspired by divine illumination was the key experience. The spiritual manifestations that accompanied it were gifts for their devotion. The idea of using any tricks to bring forth a spiritual manifestation, whether through rapping, lifting tables, or automatic writing, was offensive.

As long as the Shakers could insulate themselves from the rest of the world, their spirituality thrived. But as they felt the need to reenter the world for work, medical care, and education, the shaking started to disappear. And as they attempted to keep spiritual expression under control, the spiritual gifts faded away. Ralph Waldo Emerson gives one of the best explanations for the decline of shaking and quaking:

> The fiery reformer embodies his aspiration in some rite or covenant, and he and his friends cleave to the form and lose the aspiration. The Quaker has established Quakerism, the Shaker has established his monastery and his dance; and although each prates of spirit, there is no spirit, but repetition, which is anti-spiritual.[27]

The sociology of religion is familiar with how spirited experience or "charisma" can cool down and transform itself to ordered rituals. Max Weber called this process the "routinization of charisma." Charismatic (or ecstatic) authority and primacy are then handed over to rational-legal legitimacy. For shaking ecstatics, "the spirit is immediately present," while for institutionalized churches, "the spirit is remote" and mediated by the institution. In other words, the ecstatic experiences become domesticated and formulated.

This movement from passion and enthusiasm to calcified protocol and ritual is exactly what Emerson described. As the Shakers and Quakers brought too much order upon their spontaneous expressions of wild spirituality, the rigid routines emerged, suffocating spirited presence. Facing both internal pressure to keep ecstatic expression under control and external pressure to be accepted and trusted by outsiders for reasons of commercial and social exchange, the constituents began to establish constraints over their free expression.

Furthermore, as this expression took written form, whether as descriptions of spiritual performances at a worship service or transcriptions of a medium claiming to speak for a spirit, the texts became implicit guides and enforcers of particular practices and meanings. The authority of text stepped in, and its power took precedence over inspiration. In other words, the spontaneous explosions of spiritual energy gave way to recipes prescribed by textual (and oral) proclamations. The earliest Quakers had feared the way in which text and speech could diminish access to direct mystical experience. They originally didn't want other people's words to interfere with divine contact, to the extent that some of them downplayed the importance of the Bible.

What we learn from the Shakers and Quakers is that when we remove ourselves from outside constraints, doing so in a structure-free space, anything can happen. If there is a faithful expectation that the spirit will manifest itself, ecstatic body expression is almost certain to follow. As the body and imagination learn to be free in expressing spirited delight, there is a wide array of movements and vocalizations that may be spontaneously performed.

The Bushman tradition is familiar with many of these forms of ecstatic expression. However, Bushmen do not exhibit such a wide array of expression that we found with the Shakers and Quakers. They most likely would regard such elaboration as a distraction from going deeper into the ecstatic experience. You don't see them rolling on the ground or jumping up and down. If people go berserk, running into the wild, the others catch them, calm them down, and refocus their efforts. They favor a disciplined focus upon what I have described as the pumping of ecstatic energy up their body. They still enter into visions and revelations, but the imaginings are not given any over-importance. Since their culture is free of written texts, they are freer to move on to the next shamanic experience in the following week's dance.

Unlike that of the Quakers and Shakers, Bushman shaking, for the most part, has been respected on the African continent. Other tribal cultures are familiar with shaking and trembling, as they are featured expressions of their traditional doctors and many of their own ecstatic dances. A strong Bushman shaker is sincerely and respectfully acknowledged, and sometimes feared. He is not subject to the ridicule and punishment that the Quakers and Shakers had to endure. For thousands of years, Bushman shamans have been able to shake without outside interference. This has helped protect their shake.

The Bushman shamans are regarded as "shamans" only when they shake. When they are not shaking, they are essentially the same as everyone else. Bushman shamans are never given any inappropriate importance in the way that Mother Ann and George Fox were adulated. For the community, it is the experience of shaking, rather than the shaker, that is honored. People, ideas, and visions get leveled to the same ground in Bushman culture. However, the songs and the energy aroused by them are exalted and kept alive for the spiritual nourishment of every person.

Part of the reason that the Quakers stopped quaking and the Shakers stopped shaking was because they and outside observers took the Shakers and the shaking (and the Quakers and the quaking) too seriously. The practitioners thought they were being used as the true voices of God, while outsiders, equally serious, thought they saw true signs of mental illness or evil. What was taking place was simply and profoundly a realization of ecstatic joy, arguably the peak experience of life. The spirit made them drunk, but did so in a way that inspired them to live good lives. No matter how wise or inspiring a vision or spiritual gift might be, it too could lead to the dampening of future spontaneous spiritual expression if others believed they should replicate it. The purposeful aiming toward a particular form of spiritual expression easily short-circuited the spontaneity required for its vitality. One of the protections the Shakers used against inflating the importance of any vision or revelation was their introduction of the fool's song and dance. Had this been more honored and practiced more frequently, perhaps there would have been a tempering of the processes that routinized their texts, understandings, and practices.

They also may have resisted the routinization of their spirit if they had learned to channel the shaking energy into a more concentrated form (such as the Bushman pump) that would have taken them deeper into ecstasy, going past the spiritual/spiritualist gifts, while opening the heavens to greater epiphanies. There were times when Shakers would calibrate their ecstatic experience by turning it toward the dance. They were able to harness the energy of the jerks and other wild movements and move them into unique choreographies. Their dancing didn't necessarily serve to amplify the ecstatic currents, as it does with the Bushman shaman's pumping dance, but rather brought highly energized movement into a stabilized form of expression.

The most profound experiences are unspeakable and impossible to convey. These were the founding experiences that some of their earliest elders felt when their hearts were opened by a great divine love. Without the ongoing presence and renewal of this big love, the ecstatic gatherings too easily turned into carnivals of the spirit and spiritual materialism, the collection of more and more spiritual or spiritualist experiences.

Afraid of sexuality and prohibiting touch, the Shakers and Quakers never learned the value of shaking together with skin on skin. They must have longed to touch one another in these states of ecstasy. Their religions were handicapped by the inner battles that fought the natural desire to touch and be touched. Without touch, the experiences became too easily privatized and overtaken by imagination, rather than serving to empower relationship and the intimate expression of connection.

If there had been less attachment to visions and imaginary gifts, more levity, and more tactile contact with one another, the souls of the Shakers and Quakers might have lifted higher into the spiritual sky and their feet might have sunk more deeply into the earth. Since they did not let go of the weight of their spiritual materialism, it was only a matter of time before they crashed to the ground.

The taboo against full ecstatic expression of the human body is nothing mysterious or difficult to understand. When people enter into wild experience, they feel and look out of control. In this space, the socially established laws, rules, mores, and officiating hierarchies have no authority. It should be no surprise that most shaking and quaking has historically been associated with the oppressed, whether they are the sons and daughters of cobblers and blacksmiths or slaves and sharecroppers. The oppressed find that shaking is a medicine for the suffering of the human spirit. It sets them free and opens the doors to the kingdoms of bliss.

The shake comes as a great liberator to people in poverty, powerlessness, and suffering. It is what every religion has brought to the world. When people feel and express their deepest freedom, the surrounding social institutions will do everything they can to suppress the liberating spirit, covering it with an institutional shell and setting up explanations, routines, and monitors to bring everyone back into control. Instead of having a spirited music and dance of free expression, the context of music changes to serve the greedy and powerful elite.

For a while, the Quakers and Shakers quaked and shook forth a spiritual freedom that transformed anyone whose heart was open to receive their ecstatic gifts. In spite of their subsequent shortcomings and the eventual loss of their ecstatic expression, they showed the world that the gods await our being filled with a holy fire that can heal and recast our lives. These quaking and shaking devotees demonstrated that anyone—child, adult, or elder—can be shaken into the ecstasies that inspire and transform. Their very names—Shakers and Quakers—give testimony to the presence of shaking medicine.

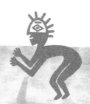

5
EXPERIENCE VERSUS IDEOLOGY

Spiritual Dilemmas in the Northwest

This chapter will examine the shaking practices of the American Indian Shakers of the Pacific Northwest, who had no association with the New England Shakers. As we did with the Quakers and the Shakers, we will compare their practices to the ecstatic ways of the Kalahari Bushmen. Here we will ponder how systems of belief influence the organization of shaking conduct. Does it matter what one believes, or can one simply shake and quake without allegiance to any religion or metaphysical theory? The hindrance and contribution of theoretical understanding to the shaking process will be further examined and challenged. I will argue that shaking bodies help loosen the grip of totalizing grand theories and literalism while encouraging deeper appreciation of whole-bodied wisdom.

I will retell the story that opened this book, this time with more detail. It began with Mary Slocum's shaking. It is the winter of 1882–1883, and an Indian logger from Puget Sound, Squ-sacht-un, known to Euro-Americans as John Slocum, has become very ill. His family pronounces his death while his brother, Jack, dispatches a canoe to Olympia with an order for a coffin. John Slocum's niece, Nancy George, a small girl at the time, is an eyewitness to his recovery from the presumed state of death. Her words were reported by Jean Todd Fredson:

> I am in the room with my aunt. My uncle's body is on a table. Outside are many Indian friends—they cry—they are very sad. In the room I sit in a corner with my aunt. She is very sad. She tells me not to look at the table but I do. I see his toes move. I tell my aunt. She says, "Don't look! Don't look!" And she will not look. But I can't help looking. After a while I see his hand move. I tell my aunt but she is too scared to look. But I look again and I see his head move. Then he sits up. Now when I tell my aunt, she looks. She sees he is alive again. She says for me to go out and tell the people to come in.
>
> When they come in John Slocum talks to them. He tells them to get down on their knees and pray. They have never prayed. He has never prayed. But he tells them that he has learned to pray up in the beautiful country, where he has been. In this country he had seen nice flowers, clear streams, and he talked with the Big Father. The Big Father has said to him, "This is not your time—go back—your people need you."[1]

This story is very similar to the experience that strong Bushman shamans have. The Bushmen experience traveling to a sky village where they meet the Sky God. There, they are taught something and encouraged to go back and help the community. The words the Sky God tells the Bushman shaman are practically identical to what John Slocum heard: "This is not your time to stay—go back—the people need you."

When John Slocum regained consciousness, he told his friends and neighbors that he needed a church built in ten days, and it was built. He said that the Big Father was going to bring a new medicine for the Indian people. As he waited for the new medicine, he started a new religion called Slocum tum-tum. A year later he became very sick again. This time his wife, Mary Slocum, who was a strong believer in his new faith, went to a stream (some reports say a beach) and started to pray. Her hands began to shake and then her whole body was shaking. As an eye-witness report from Annie James, John Slocum's sister-in-law, testified:

> [Mary Slocum] went to the beach in grief, while there she collapsed, and for some time she was out, and when she came to, she was trembling from her feet to the crown of her head. In other words she was under the power of God, the Holy Spirit was in charge of her. That was the first born of the so-called Indian Shaker Church.[2]

Everyone who touched Mary Slocum started shaking. When the shaking resulted in the recovery of John Slocum, he announced that "the shake" was the new medicine. On that day, Slocum tum-tum became the Shaker religion of the American Indians.

The ingredients for the Indian Shakers' ceremonial practice were born the moment Mary Slocum first shook. As she shook in front of her sick husband, she asked people to bring her a wooden cross. She started singing the first Indian Shaker songs and asked for handbells to be brought and rung. Dancing in a circle, she spontaneously performed what became known as the structure of the Indian Shaker worship and healing rituals. When she gave the shake to her husband, he was surprised to see his hands trembling and his body shaking. In this spontaneous ecstatic display, their religion was born.

A typical Indian Shaker meeting had a small table in the middle of the room holding a wooden cross, candles, and bells. As bell ringers stood in the center and clanged the bells, people would circle them, allowing their bodies and arms to wildly shake. Those not shaking stood against the walls of the room. Those who shook proceeded to dance and stomp their feet in rhythm with the ringing bells. Chants and songs were voiced, and from time to time, some shakers would pause near someone and pass their hands over that person's body, trying to remove illness and sin. A circle of shaking bodies moved around and around the bell ringers in a ring dance that inspired ecstatic fervor.

Albert Reagan described their worship as jumping up and down to the time of the ringing bells and communally sung music. He characterized their shaking as "[t]he quivering, trembling, twisting, writhing hands [that] wave, whirl, gyrate in all directions till the scene reminds one much of the demons in the 'inferno' dancing over a lost soul."

Their dance, though somewhat similar to that of the New England Shakers, arose independently of the latter. Ober provides a description of the Indian Shaker dance:

> Soon the dancers form a wide circle. . . . The rhythmic clang of bells, the wild singing, the regular thud of heavy feet grows faster and faster, wilder and wilder, as the ardor of the worshippers increases. With upturned introspective faces, closed eyes, clasped hands, all seem oblivious to any outward thing, but somehow keep perfect step and time, avoiding all obstacles. They begin to gesticulate, and to me, every motion is full of meaning, and seldom devoid of grace. Some extend their arms, with waving motions, as if swimming through seas of ecstasy; others reach upwards, their hands outspread as if to grasp some occult power; some stroke and brush their bodies, ending each movement with an outward, downward fling, as if removing accumulations of sins; some with intent, absorbed countenances, in attitudes of petition, are lost in devotion. . . .
>
> The scene baffles description. More and more violent grows the dance, the noise, the whirling figures. Twirling like dervishes, weaving in and out of the circle, they dance. . . . Rough, sin-scarred men are transfigured, their faces shining with some mysterious inward power, their gnarled hands outstretched as if to take hold of the very God Himself. Young men and women lithely spring and dance, totally oblivious to sense or sex, completely dominated by that strange ecstasy. Suddenly the "shaking" comes upon someone, every nerve, muscle, and limb shaken in a manner impossible to describe. . . . They claim it is an answer to prayer, and is the power of God, coming into their lives.[3]

As in other shaking traditions, music drives the ecstatic expression. The Indian Shakers believe their songs are delivered from heaven and come to them through dreams or when they shake. Sometimes they sing only a few words and then change to repeating the sound *hai, hai.* As in their previous shamanic culture, the song gave spiritual power to the Indian Shakers and to their ceremony. It was common for them to call a song "a help."

As they sang, the loud rhythm of a bell started at a slow beat and then gradually escalated. They started at around sixty to seventy beats per minute and then went up to two hundred fifty per minute.[4] When the rhythm reached a peak, the leader typically began another song, again starting at a slower beat and gradually building up the rate until another climax was reached. This is the rhythmic cycle that accompanied escalating shaking in a healing or worship service.

In addition to their worship services, the Indian Shakers held meetings in their homes to heal the sick. Called "night work," this is where the remnants of their former shamanic ways were most evident. In a frenzied state, they would try to rub the illness out of a person's body. Marian Smith provides an account of early Indian Shakers who healed:

> Alice James and I used to go around and shake to cure people. . . .
> We shook one night until one o'clock and then I walked four miles
> home. The next day the patient felt better. When we came the fifth
> day, the patient was sitting up and he felt better. This night we
> shook until two o'clock and they asked us to stay there the rest of
> the night. When we had started, the patient could barely whisper he
> was so weak. Now he was up and about and he got well.[5]

For the Indian Shakers, healing typically involves three patterns of movement: brushing, rubbing, and the push-and-pull. Brushing is the most common movement. It usually involves a fanning motion of the hands over the body's surface while the feet stomp. Rubbing involves the shaker resting his or her hand on the exact spot where the sickness is located. At that site, the shaking becomes stronger as the hands rub it with a cleansing motion. Eventually the hands cup and clench as if catching the sickness. The sickness is then released with a jerking motion of the hands, usually upward toward the heavens. The push-and-pull technique requires the most work because it involves heavy physical exertion on the patient's body. It may involve the participation of several healers at the same time, and in its most dramatic form, the patient is shaken quite aggressively.

The Bushman shaman's fluttering hands also touch a person's body. After shaking it for a while, a shaman may rub the body and appear to collect the illness before throwing it away into the air. Like the Indian Shakers, Bushman shamans may hold people and shake them wildly. They usually do so by embracing the person with a huge shaking hug, or several shamans may administer shaking all at once. Sometimes the shamans fall on top of each other, shaking as a huge mass while lying on the ground. Here they heal and empower one another to continue the healing work with the community.

One could not be an Indian Shaker until one received "the shake," which was believed to be a gift from God. The shake restored, recharged, revitalized, regenerated, soothed, and brought about a heightened sense of well-being. Under its influence, the Indians could have visions, be clairvoyant, see into the spiritual nature of things, and diagnose and cure sickness. When a person decided to become an Indian Shaker, the other Indian Shakers helped the person get the shake. The head person of a church put the shake, called "God's medicine," into the hands of the candidate, while the other members formed a circle around them. The bells were rung as everyone started shaking. This continued until the candidate started to shake.

There were times when a shaker may have wanted to get more strength. He or she would then request "a shake" for the purpose of getting more spiritual energy. The congregation would circle the recipient, who held a lit candle. The bells were rung as the group started shaking and transferring the shake to the person. They shook and marched in one direction and, after a while, turned and marched in the other direction. When the person felt strengthened, he or she would blow out the candle and the ceremony would stop.

When people got the shaking power, they typically demonstrated increased physical activity, "such as louder stamping, shaking of the hands and body, a taut facial expression with the eyes closed, and much perspiration."[6] In the beginning of the religion, all kinds of miracles were reported. Some people even tried to fly or walk upon water. That's how ecstatic the shaking made them feel.

Seen from the perspective of local history, shaking did not first appear to the Northwest Indians through Mary Slocum's initial bout of ecstatic movements. It already had been part of the healing ceremony called the Spirit-Canoe. Along these lines, the anthropologist T. T. Waterman proposed that the shaking in the Spirit-Canoe ceremony was "the exact counterpart of the modern Shaker exercise" and that "for generations. . . . there [had] been 'shaking phenomena connected with the [Spirit-Canoe] performances.'"[7]

In his article "The Paraphernalia of the Duwamish 'Spirit-Canoe' Ceremony," Waterman described the body shaking associated with medicine men who held "power objects":

[T]he power is accompanied by certain peculiar motor disturbances. The Indians say that the objects used are entered by the "power," and in this condition they quiver, jump about, and drag around the people who try to hold them. The psychological explanation undoubtedly is that there is an expectancy of a certain definite pattern in the minds of the performers, who get the shaking visitation and contribute the resultant quivering and jerking to the objects which they hold . . . [the quivering seizures] occur also in the spirit-canoe ceremony. . . . The owner of the power may announce, after a time, "My power will now enter those drum poles." The poles "of themselves" then begin to shake. The men can scarcely hold them.[8]

Waterman's point is that quite a few traditional Indian ceremonies are believed to involve power objects that come to life. The power of the objects is displayed by the way they tremble and shake. What is more likely going on is that the shaman's body is shaking, thereby causing the object to shake. The shaman might say the opposite: The powerful shaking of the object causes the shaman to shake.

For almost all shamans, trembling and shaking are signs that contact has been made with spiritual power. The shaking medicine man was often misunderstood by missionaries and outside government authorities, mistakenly diagnosed as someone possessed by evil spirits. Accordingly, the shaking had to go underground and be hidden. In addition, the frenetic and wild shaking body may have been too much for all people to see, Indians included. If this was the case, it would be natural that ceremonies began to take place in the dark, or a way was found to cover the shaman's shaking body. For the Cree, Ojibway, and others, the "shaking tent" ceremony was one of the most powerful healing rites. A medicine man would enter a specially made tent and call forth the spirits, and then the tent would begin shaking, wildly moving back and forth. Early observations suggest that when the medicine man went inside the tent, he would hold on to the poles of the structure as his body shook in an ecstatic fit. Anthropologist A. Irving Hallowell wrote this account in 1942:

> The conventional position which the conjurer [shaman] is supposed to assume in the lodge is one of the commonly made sitting postures. The knees rest on the ground and the buttocks against the heels. It is the ordinary posture of a canoeman paddling in the bow; but in the conjuring lodge the upper part of the body is bent forward until the head almost touches the ground. . . . [w]ith his right hand the conjurer grabs one of the upright poles not far from the ground. As soon as he does so he "feels something strange," I was told, and the structure begins to vibrate.[9]

Did the tent shake the medicine man or did the man shake the tent? More generally, do the spirits shake the human being, the tent, and the sacred objects, or does the ecstatic shaking body bring forth the spirited performance?

One of the last great medicine men, Albert Lightning, from Alberta,

Canada, used to shake when he healed. His apprentice, Dave Gehue, a blind Micmac medicine man, also shook. Dave said to me when I attended one of his shaking tent ceremonies, "Yes, in the old days the medicine men and women used to shake. That's when they had the power. Now the shaking is almost gone. There are few medicine people with strong power. For me, it's simple: no shake, no shaman." One can easily argue that the shaking body and trembling hands of medicine people were always present in the traditional ceremonies of North America. The appearance of the Indian Shakers was simply one example of the shake moving from one ceremony to another. In the same way that the shake can be passed from one person to another, it can move across ceremonial situations and practices.

The Indian Shakers began in the 1880s, a time when traditional Indian religious practice was forbidden by the U.S. government. Government agents had banned all traditional forms of Indian doctoring. With Shakerism, the Indians were able to move some of the ecstatic, visionary, and shamanic aspects of their old ways into an acceptable form. With this religion, "anyone with faith in a new power could do the things only shamans could do before."[10] Rather than being possessed or related to a "guardian spirit," now one could be solely possessed and/or influenced by God, the Big Father. Judge James Wickersham, of Tacoma, Washington, although a dubious character, successfully fought to get the Indian Shaker church legally accepted as a religion, allowing the Indians to practice an ecstatic form of worship.

Similarly, Gunther concluded that "the appeal of the new religion was much greater after shaking was included in the ritual, for its activity was akin to the procedure of the shaman, as well as to the outward expression of spirit possession." In this respect, Mary Slocum is as responsible for the religion as her husband because she brought the shake into it. As soon as word traveled about the shake, the religion spread like wildfire, moving from Squaxin Island both south and north, including Oregon, Washington, California, and Canada. The curing power of the shake and its spirited expression in worship services were what principally attracted the Indian people.

Albert Reagan, in 1908, wrote that the Indian Shaker "watchword" was "Do good to those who do good to you and get 'even' with those who mistreat you." He implied that Indian Shakers, like their medicine men, were able to "take care of things," whether that involved healing or protection of loved ones. In the beginning, some Indian Shakers were accused of shamanic "doctoring." The court records of the Tulalip Indians show charges against shakers for "doctoring" in 1902, 1904, and 1906. They were accused of bringing harm, even murder, to others in their efforts to heal. These claims were most likely due to the missionaries and government agents wanting to stop the spread of the Indian Shaker church, seeing it as no different from old shamanic practices.

Most Indian Shakers renounced the harmful practices of their native shamans (causing sickness and death in others) while believing in the shamans' good practices—the power to heal. For the most part, they singularly focused on bringing God's message into their hearts. They prayed sincerely, sometimes for as long as several days, to receive "God's gift." They waited patiently to receive a divine message that would help them live a good spiritual life.

John Slocum had been quite a rascal before his resurrection experience. Described as a "bad" man who couldn't stop gambling, swearing, drinking, or cheating, his deathlike experience changed his ways. In Slocum's own words: "All at once I saw a shining light, a great light, trying my soul. I looked at my own body and saw it was dead. Angels told me to look back and see my body. I did and saw it lying down."[11] Slocum claimed to have met an angel at the gates to heaven who told him that he couldn't be held fully responsible for his wicked ways because he, like other Indians, was unable to read the Bible. The angel made him a prophet and told him to provide spiritual leadership for the other Indians. He was instructed to return and lead others away from a sinful life. As a consequence, members of the Indian Shaker church weren't allowed to drink or gamble.

Like other shaking practices that came on the American scene, the Indians' shaking religion was not well received by the local authorities.

As Sarah Ober reported, "It met with great opposition from the Government officials, missionaries, and white people, and every means was used to check, or to stamp it out. The leaders were imprisoned, persecuted, ridiculed, discouraged in every way, but nothing could obliterate their faith."[12]

One of the Indian Shakers, Big John of Skokomish, rode on horseback through Olympia with his arms extended like the crucified Christ. He rode in with his wife and about fifty enthusiastic followers. Big John was immediately arrested and jailed by the police in the same way the English had imprisoned a Quaker preacher for blasphemy nearly a hundred years before for riding an ass into town while accompanied by a group of women.

Keep in mind that the nineteenth century was filled with spirited religious expression. Each new practice borrowed and built upon the practices that had come before. In the Pacific Northwest, some of these religious orientations leaned more toward traditional Native culture, while others leaned more toward mixing old ways with Christian beliefs. It was also common for people to participate in several kinds of religion. For instance, some Indian Shakers were also Coast Salish spirit dancers. For them, the "Indian Way" and Christian beliefs were complementary. Others, however, believed that one was either a Christian or a lost soul. But for those who tried both ways, they found that "people who participate in both the spirit dancing and the Shake have equal facility in becoming entranced in either setting."[13]

The shaking of the Indian Shakers was probably passed to them from the ceremonies of the Spirit-Canoe, the Power Sing, and Coast Salish spirit dancing, among others. And from the Indian Shakers, other ceremonies received the shake. These might include the rites of the Feather Cult and even the historic Ghost Dance. With regard to the latter, Mooney writes that "[i]ndeed, there is good reason to believe that the Paiute messiah himself, and through him, all the apostles of the Ghost dance, have obtained their knowledge of hypnotic secrets from the 'Shakers' of Puget Sound."[14]

The Ghost Dance was an ecstatic circle dance that spread throughout

Indian country. Started in western Nevada by a Paiute Indian named Wokova, it involved a dance that brought on trembling and shaking, collapsing to the ground, and visionary experiences. Inspired by a vision received during a solar eclipse, Wokova believed that the dance provided a way for the ancestral spirits, the spirits of the dead from the spirit world, to come back and provide guidance and inspiration. Wokova regarded himself as a messiah whose job was to prepare the Indians for salvation. He believed that the white people would be buried and the buffalo would return. This would take place while the Indians were suspended in the heavens. When they came back to Earth, their ancestors would join them.

Slocum, Wokova, and other originators of Indian religious movements began with a revelation and prophetic experience. The subsequent power associated with their ceremonial performances involved trembling, shaking, and further vision. In Wokova's case, the name of the Ghost Dance was given by white people who heard about the Indians' beliefs in a resurrection that was followed by a reunion with their dead ancestors. Each Indian group had a different name for the dance. Wokova encouraged the dance to take place as often as possible, believing that it would hasten the arrival of the new world.

As the Ghost Dance movement increased, the government agents panicked and asked for troops to quell the "pernicious system of religion." Although one agent, Valentine McGillycuddy, recommended that the Indians be allowed to continue their dance, the government banned the dance, as it had all other traditional ceremonies. Eventually, the horrible massacre of Wounded Knee resulted, in which troops slaughtered women and children for dancing it in South Dakota.

Once again, a dance that promoted shaking was feared and attacked, as if it could do harm to the rest of the world. The Indians at Wounded Knee weren't the only ecstatic, shaking dancers to be attacked by an angry mob. Many years earlier, in 1810, at Turtle Creek, Ohio, a mob of five hundred armed men, accompanied by two thousand supporters, attacked the local Shaker community. They did so because the Shakers had "made a shipwreck of our faith, and turned aside to an old woman's fables."[15] Yes, shaking dances are dangerous—they bring forth an experience of freedom and hope for a better world that threatens the privileged classes. The Ghost Dance was not that different from what the Quakers, Shakers, Indian Shakers, and many other ecstatic groups had performed. Mooney writes:

> As to the dance itself, with its scenes of intense excitement, spasmodic action, and physical exhaustion even to unconsciousness, such manifestations have always accompanied religious upheavals among primitive peoples, and are not entirely unknown among ourselves. In a country which produces magnetic healers, shakers, trance mediums, and the like, all these things may very easily be paralleled without going very far away from home.[16]

An Oglala Sioux Indian named George Sword wrote a description and explanation of the Ghost Dance in the Teton Dakota dialect, which was translated in Mooney's historic Smithsonian report as follows:

> [P]eople partaking in dance would get crazy and die, then the messiah is seen and all the ghosts. When they die they see strange things, they see their relatives who died long before. They saw these things when they died in ghost dance and came to life again. The person dancing becomes dizzy and finally drop[s] dead, and the first thing they saw is an eagle comes to them and carried them to where the messiah is with his ghosts. . . .
>
> The persons in the ghost dancing are all joined hands. A man stands and then a woman, so in that way forming a very large circle. They dance around in the circle in a continuous time until some of them become so tired and overtired that they become crazy and finally drop as though dead, with foams in mouth all wet by perspiration.[17]

Ghosts could also be seen by some of the more spiritually gifted Indian Shakers. Ghosts were regarded as capable of holding human feelings, attitudes, and needs while in another dimension. Some, but not all

Indian Shakers, believed that ghosts, described as floating, fast-traveling fogs, could be the cause of misfortune, accidents, and sickness. As the old Salish shamans did, Indian Shakers thought that one's vital essence or soul could be kidnapped by lonely ghosts wanting companionship. When one's soul was taken by a ghost or lost due to an emotional or physical shock, these Indian Shakers searched to find the soul and place it back into the body. This was classic shamanic work. Consider this account from Roland Olson:

> Three years ago Mrs. T. S. had an operation. She grew steadily weaker and finally was taken home, near dead. . . . The third night Mrs. C. S. found her soul in the road in front of H. S.'s house. It had fallen out on the way to the hospital when the truck went over a bump. The Shakers put the soul back and every night kept up the shaking. She mended rapidly and in a year was entirely well.[18]

While shaking, the spiritually gifted Indian Shakers could see these ghosts and see the lost souls. Klan writes:

> Some shakers under [shaking] power can see the lost souls, which are light, fluffy, and "like a fog." Others are led to the soul by a thread "like a cobweb," or by an invisible guiding force. When the wayward soul is found the group restores it to the body with smoothing and patting motions.[19]

The Bushman shamans, while under the influence of shaking ecstasy, also see threads and lines that connect them to their ancestral spirits. They, too, smooth and pat the body to help restore it in their healing practices. Shaking shamans, whether from the Pacific Northwest or the Kalahari, feel an intense sense of clarity and intuitive understanding while they are being shaken. They feel that they shift from being in the thoughts of the head to being in the feelings of the heart. Shaking transforms the shaker into a heart-centered transforming agent to others.

The Bushman shamans' most powerful experience is seeing a rope hanging from the sky. When they approach it, they are lifted to the celestial village where God meets and teaches them. In 1884, Peter Heck was converted to shakerism and described his experience as follows:

> Last Saturday night my hands began to shake, and then they crossed each other and shook two hours. I was sitting on a pile of rails. Then I knelt down and shook two hours; then stood shaking three hours; then stood with my arms stretched out straight, one-half hour; then I took hold of a rope that reached to heaven, with both hands.[20]

In the beginning of the Indian Shaker religion, shaking was applied to almost every imaginable thing the shaker desired, "for fair weather, favorable winds, for success in fishing or hunting, for escape from danger or deliverance from trouble; to exorcise evil spirits, and cast out diseases, as well as for salvation from sin."[21] At that time, they shook for days and sometimes for weeks, until they became completely exhausted. The U.S. government, in an effort to control the shaking, made it illegal to shake except for several hours a week, but never past midnight! Reverend Myron Eells, a missionary in the region, wrote:

> It also became a serious question whether the constant shaking of their heads would not make some of them crazy, and from symptoms and indications it was the opinion of the agency physician, J. T. Martin, that it would do so. Accordingly, on the reservation the authority of the agent was brought to bear, and to a great extent the shaking was stopped. . . . Some at first said they could not stop shaking, but that at their prayer meetings and church services on the Sabbath their hands and heads would continue to shake in spite of themselves; but after a short time, when the excitement had died away, they found that they could stop.[22]

Other foreign cultures more familiar with shaking, such as the Bushman, Zulu, and other African traditions, recognize that a beginning shamanic initiate will shake uncontrollably for great lengths of time. Among the Zulu, the beginner is taken to a senior *sangoma,* or medicine person, who will watch over him or her for as long as it takes for the shaking to become familiar and manageable.[23] Among the Guarani Indians of South America, the spirits must be given time to "settle into the body."[24] In the case of the Indian Shakers, perhaps only the first generation of believers developed a full-blown initiation into the shaking. After their shaking settled in, the next group of converts was discouraged from the intense shaking the originators had gone through. As a result, the intensity and duration of future shaking may have lessened.

For Indian Shakers, the force or energy that shakes them was simply referred to as "their shake." They would say things like "My shake told me" or "The shake cured him." Although their shaking might appear to be uncontrolled to outside observers, the shaking of their experienced practitioners was actually stylized and patterned. Some of the body movements were spontaneous, while others fell into recognizable forms, often unique to the particular practitioner. An individual Bushman shaman or Indian Shaker is known for the way he or she shakes and moves. Each shaman or shaker may develop his or her own style of shaking. As we mentioned before, beginning shakers are all over the place. They are learning to shake in a variety of ways, but over time, the shaking starts to fit inside some recognizable forms. The forms may be ones they observed from other elders, or they may fall into place naturally without any outside influence.

Although experienced shakers' movements become stylized and patterned, we must remember that the shakers have no idea why they move and shake in a particular way. None of them receives any purposeful instruction. The Indian Shakers and Bushman shamans have never been taught how to shake or move their bodies. They only feel spontaneous, effortless motion that comes about naturally. They say that the power of God causes every shaking movement. One Indian Shaker said, "I don't know what John Slocum or Mud Bay Louis did with their hands. Nobody taught me anything. If I am right with the heavenly power it will come into my hands. I don't think what I am going to do. The power does it. Look, now, I'm a Shaker; so is my friend, George. But our hands don't go alike."[25]

As we examine the various shaking traditions, from the Kalahari to the Quakers, Shakers, Indian Shakers, and Ghost Dancers, we find we can discern some general things about shaking medicine. First, it always begins as a wild explosion of energized expression that immediately attracts followers as well as those who are ready to criticize and attack. In its initial period, every imaginable kind of experience can take place. It is a wild carnival or circus of spirited expression. Over time, the spirited expression becomes mediated by oral or written explanations, theories, and mythologies. This is when a schism starts to appear, with some practitioners going in the direction of keeping the practice as a spontaneous revelation of guidance and another group seeking textual guidance and socially sanctified forms, protocols, and rituals.

Nearly half a century from the time Mary Slocum started shaking, the Indian Shakers split in two. In 1936, William Kitsap, of Tulalip, announced that the Shakers needed the Bible. "For 24 years the word of God has been out of these Shaker Churches, and now we must get the word of God established in all churches." Another Indian Shaker added his voice to the chorus: "You can shake without it [the Bible], but you need it to know whether you are right or wrong."[26] After exalting the place of the Bible, it wasn't long before the Indian Shakers received competition from Bible-quoting Pentecostals. This worried some Indian Shaker leaders, because they didn't believe it was possible for their religion to compete and survive if it didn't allow for the inclusion of biblical authority.

On the other side of the fence, some leaders were criticized for relying too much on the Bible. Wilbur Martin, a strong advocate of the Bible, was sent to an Indian Shaker church in Siletz, Oregon. It didn't take long for the congregation to get angry with Martin for preaching "the white man's Bible." Eventually, he was carried out of the church by members of the anti-Bible group.[27]

Like the early Quakers, the Indian Shakers in the beginning days of their religion wanted only direct divine inspiration and no interference from textual authority. The Bible, for these practitioners, was largely ignored in favor of ecstatic experience. Those who kept this attitude were called Old Shake; those who began to use the Bible, which happened around 1927, were called Full Gospel. A third group, the Independents, were somewhere in the middle. They might use the Bible, but they did not force it on anyone.

The Old Shake practitioners believed that "if I prayed I would have power and be a medicine man."[28] They did not concern themselves with biblical beliefs, but placed their trust in God, Jesus, and the reality of heaven and hell. The Indian Shaker faith was arguably a way of replacing the old medicine men. The Indian Shakers' appearance made strange bedfellows of the local church authorities and the old medicine men who joined together to fight the existence of the shaking religion. However, the shake was too strong to be stopped, and the Indian Shaker became the medicine man who worked exclusively for good while warning that the old traditional medicine man would be tempted to work for evil. As one of the Shakers, Sam Yowaluch, put it:

> A good Christian is a good medicine man. A good Christian man in the dark sees a light toward God. God makes a fog—good Christian man goes straight through it to the end, like good medicine. I believe this religion. It helps poor people. Bad men can't see good— bad men can't get to heaven—can't find his way. We were sent to jail for this religion, but we will never give up.[29]

Imagine the Indian Shakers' (and Quakers' and Shakers') delight if they had known about the gnostic gospels, which hadn't been discovered when the Indian Shaker church began. The gnostic gospels emphasize "gnosis," a form of inner knowing and communicating with the divine. The Gnostics claimed that whoever "sees the Lord" through spiritual vision "can claim that his or her own authority equals, or surpasses, that of the twelve [apostles]."[30] In the Acts of John, one of the most respected gnostic texts, Jesus is described as joined with his disciples in Gethsemane just prior to being arrested. The scripture reads:

> He assembled us all, and said, "before I am delivered to them, let us sing a hymn to the Father, and so go to meet what lies before (us)."

So He told us to form a circle, holding one another's hands, and Himself stood in the middle. . . . "I will pipe, Dance all of you. . . . To the Universe belongs the Dancer. He who does not dance does not know what happens. Now if you follow my dance, see yourself in Me who is speaking and when you have seen what I do, keep silence about my mysteries. . . . I have suffered none of the things which they will say of me; even that suffering which I showed to you and to the rest in my dance, I will that it be called a mystery."

The Indian Shakers, along with the Quakers and Shakers, were natural gnostics. No shaker disputed the validity of the Bible. What they argued about was its use. Should the Bible be given a higher authority over the shake? Should it be used to interpret and shape the performance of the shake? Or should it be the other way around: allowing the power of the shake to open one's spiritual eyes and heart so that then and only then one could be in a position to receive the truth of the sacred words? Each side of the debate felt it had the absolute truth on this matter, and the Indian Shaker church began to break apart.

In this period of competitive fighting, some Indian Shakers left the church altogether and returned to the Spirit Dance of the Smokehouse (a large traditional meeting place, sometimes called a longhouse, where ceremonial practices are conducted). They were drawn there for the same reason they had been drawn to the Indian Shakers in the first place. There, they felt spiritual power, something that could deliver spiritual and physical healing. Many Indian Shakers had already been going to both Shaker and Smokehouse meetings, but when the church started arguing over the role of the Bible, some of them stopped going to the Indian Shakers altogether. For them, politics, rather than spiritual worship, had moved onto center stage. And that wasn't what they were after.

Other disagreements erupted, with arguments over whether it was a good thing to enter different spiritual communities and practices. In the beginning, there was no problem with intermingling among different houses of worship. But over time, some people said that a parishioner had to choose one over the other. Another factor came into play: As the church sought to be further institutionalized, it had to go through legal procedures to be recognized as a church, enabling it to have tax benefits and the like. Church members became more business-minded, and this made them less tolerant of any competition. This, too, may have pulled them farther away from the spontaneous shaking that originally started the movement. Ober further describes how some of the Indian Shaker churches gradually moved toward a recognizable institutional form:

> But Shakerism has gradually eliminated much of the ancient super-stitions, and has been slowly evolving into a Christian religion. Each year it gains some new practice, some valuable precept from Christianity. Within a few years the Shakers have discovered baptism, and made it a part of their church doctrine. They now have their own Bishop.[31]

The shamanic traditions that preceded the Indian Shakers were also challenged with similar issues. They, too, advocated the importance of certain ideas and beliefs, and in so doing, their shaking spiritual power was modified and constrained to conform to a received view of things. A shamanic culture is as susceptible to the forces of institutionalization as that of a sect or church. Eliade's distinction between ecstatic shamans and ritualist shamans points to this. The ritualist easily loses the spiritual power that the original ecstatic created. When a shamanic leader dreams a ceremony, its first performances pour forth intense spiritual energy and excitement. After the ceremony has been performed hundreds or thousands of times and taught to others, certain preconceptions about form and understanding get concretized, resulting in the ceremony surrendering to the constraints of orthodoxy. The ecstatic's spirited performance then turns into the ritualist's routine.

To keep the spirit alive, a culture must have a loose enough form that allows for constant modification, individual contribution, and surprise. Bushman culture does this quite well. Megan Biesele notes of the Bushman tradition, "[T]he power of the religion itself may lie in its having provided an amendable, growing form to which individuals, working idiosyncratic experience into concerted social understanding, can add meaning."[32] What this means is that although there are some basic ideas that remain relatively stable in Bushman culture, each shaman's visions and experiences are allowed as legitimate, even if they contradict someone else's experience. Because of their acknowledgment of the ever-changing trickster, they expect a shaman's experience to be shape shifting, including the understandings, ideas, and metaphors.

When a culture demands homogenization of its ideas and practices, its spirited expression, particularly shaking, starts to die out. When the Indian Shakers were comfortable with their members going in and out of different ceremonial atmospheres, the spirit was alive and well. When they gave in to sole reliance upon one form and one book, the institutional forces started to dampen the charismatic impulse. As mental chatter, public debate, and textual engagement became more dominant, the quaking stopped.

What would it be like to quake and shake without any beliefs? Can there be such a state of mind? After all, believing that you have no beliefs is itself a unique belief. Even if one is agnostic, there is arguably going to be present some form of implicit understanding and underlying epistemology (way of knowing). Similarly, the contemporary religion-less packaging of neo-shamanism is basically a re-dressing or repackaging of the shamanic impulse into the religion of science, or scientism, in which ideas like sonic-driving and cortical stimulation provide new meaning for spirited experience. As the Indian Shakers once took the old shamanic ways and Christianized them, neo-shamans take the old practices and scientize them.

When a mystery is reduced to convenient explanation, whether religious, psychological, or scientific, it loses its ability to evoke spirited expression. After all, when you think that you understand what is going on, you take out the mystery. More accurately, you lose your relationship with mystery and the feeling of awe that accompanies it. Without mystery, there is less room for inspiration. Things have been explained away, and prediction rather than spontaneity now rules the performance.

When the old shamanic ways of the Pacific Northwest became too easily clichéd by their routine ways of practice and interpretation, the Indian Shakers came along and added some mystery and a new form of minimalist interpretation. There was room for the spirit to play. As the Bible became more present and rigidly interpreted, along with prescribed orderings of their liturgy, the shaking didn't go on for days and weeks, as it had in the beginning. But when the parishioners went back and forth to different ceremonial houses, the spiritual power of both places was lifted. Because the practitioners were not overly constrained by one or the other, neither setting had a rigid hold on the shaking or the hermeneutics.

The lesson here is that the spirit must be free to roam if it is to survive and thrive. Its house must be open and spacious enough for movement, and its ceremonial structures must be receptive and adaptive to improvisational change. Most importantly, sacred books and oral stories must be read with the intent to inspire the bringing forth of mystery and ecstatic expression, rather than being stern gatekeepers, single-minded judges, and fixed interpreters of the experience. Inspiration must override understanding and freedom must prevail over rigid structure.

When the shake is truly valued and protected, it will help keep the spirit alive. Through shaking, the tight grip of any totalizing ideology is loosened. Shaking is a medicine to help prevent the hardening of conceptual categories. It keeps our vessel open for the spirit to flow through. As the Lakota medicine man Fools Crow put it, we need to be a hollow tube for the Great Spirit to pass through. Shaking helps keep us a hollow tube and an empty vessel. And finally, it is not only our bodies that need to be shaken; our words and meanings must also shake. When the spirit moves through us, everything will shake—our understandings, actions, and experiences. Shake in order to set free your mind, body, and soul.

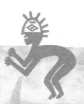

6

HARNESSING THE SHAKE

Spiritual Traveling in the Caribbean

The Spiritual Baptists of St. Vincent (formerly called the St. Vincent Shakers, though having no connection to the New England Shakers) practice a shamanic blend of Christianity and African spiritual traditions. Today, some prefer to call themselves "The Converted," while others use the term "Spiritual Baptists." They represent one of the most active shamanic cultures in the world, and access to spiritual and healing knowledge is open to all of its practitioners. I studied and participated in their tradition and will describe how some of their ways enhance shaking medicine. In particular, the deepening of spirituality through ceremonial participation, commitment to a tradition, and fasting rituals can empower the therapeutic ability to shake. I will also further our discussion of how shaking is a means of bringing forth spiritual vision and luminous experience.

St. Vincent is one of the Windward Islands, located one hundred ninety miles north of Trinidad and one hundred miles south of Barbados. It is lush with vegetation and contains a volcano, Mt. Soufrière, whose previous eruptions have caused extensive damage and loss of life. Unlike the mix of African religion and Catholicism that characterized the formation of Santería in Cuba, Candomblé in Brazil, and Vodou in Haiti, Shakerism among the Spiritual Baptists in the Caribbean island of St. Vincent was a blend of African traditions with the Protestant church, particularly the Methodist church. Henney wrote, "Shakers say that John and Charles Wesley were the originators of their religion."[1] Certainly, the fervent shaking of John Wesley would have been a good match for the shaking practices of the ecstatic African religions.

In the earliest appearances of the Spiritual Baptists (then called Shakers), the practice was rather wild, with shaking bodies and loud shouting. It caused such a commotion that it frightened the governor's horse, causing him to fall to the ground. Governor Gideon Murray ordered the faith illegal. In 1912, an ordinance was passed "to render illegal the practice of 'Shakerism' as indulged in the colony of St. Vincent," saying that "a certain ignorant section of the inhabitants" was gathering and carrying on with practices "which tend to exercise a pernicious and demoralizing effect upon said inhabitants." In a speech made by the colonial administrator who advocated the ordinance, he described shaking as a "relic of barbarism."

Persecution had actually begun with the raiding and destruction of the early Methodist ministers' homes, and many years later, those found shaking were sent to prison. The ordinance was not repealed until 1965. In the early days, they were called everything from Clap Hands to barefoot religion, candlelight religion, Believers, the Penitent, and Tieheads (because of the bands they wrap around their heads), while a few were named Jumpers.

In spite of constant persecution and lack of respect, the Spiritual Baptists physically survived and spiritually thrived. Today, the Spiritual Baptists comprise an active community of spiritual practitioners. Their prayer houses, or praise houses, are spread throughout the island, and meetings, often lasting four to five hours, are held regularly. The shaking religion was also developed in Trinidad, where practitioners were originally called Shouters, but today are similarly regarded as Spiritual Baptists. Other Caribbean groups that closely resemble their practice are the Revivalists of Jamaica and the Jordanites of Guyana. Haitian Vodou is also similar to the Spiritual Baptist religion. Although they are not historically related to the New England Shakers or the Indian

Shakers, "the practices of the Converted [Spiritual Baptists] bear such strong similarity to the Shakers of the Northwest that one cannot fail to notice."[2]

In the beginning days of the Spiritual Baptists, it was sometimes difficult to separate the African from the Christian forms of ecstatic expression. As with the Indian Shakers of the Pacific Northwest, concern developed over how to keep different traditions separate. Some Spiritual Baptists (including those from Trinidad) didn't want the two traditions and gods to mix. They developed a liturgical structure that began with a time for purification, spiritually cleaning the praise house to be free of any unwelcome spirits. They rang bells, prayed, and sprinkled water in every corner and entrance of the house. The cleansing practice, called "surveying," still takes place.

After the place had been spiritually cleaned, they began hymns and prayers that purposefully avoided the awakening or stirring of the spirit. This part of the liturgy was called the "cool period." After the place had been made ready and everyone felt certain that only the spirit of God would enter, the songs changed. Now the Holy Ghost was invited into the church. Things immediately became "hot," and all the familiar forms of shaking and quaking took place. Grunts, shouts, animal cries, hand clapping, drumming, rhythmic hyperventilated breathing called 'doption, and speaking in tongues would then occur. When the hot zone was completed, things cooled down again. Approximately sixty to seventy percent of a service would be cool, while the remaining portion was spiritually hot.

For the St. Vincent way of shaking, entry into the hot zone can be seen as taking place in three phases: First, they connect with the spirit, and the spirit starts to do its work. The shaker's body begins to feel somewhat out of control. Body movements and sounds take on a random appearance and are not patterned or entrained to a rhythm. In this first phase, there are spontaneous jerks, shivering, trembling, unexpected shouts, sobs, hisses, and unintelligible sounds.

The second phase takes place when the spirit is believed to be moving you in a strong way. Now the spirit is in control, and it provides the deepest ecstatic experiences. Body movements and sounds are rhythmical, patterned, and often in synch with those of the group. Strong overbreathing called 'doption, alternately sucking air and releasing it with a grunting sound, takes place. The body may bend forward from the waist with knees slightly bent, assuming the same posture as a dancing Bushman shaman. This is the time when a shaker can touch the candle flame and not be burned, similar to the Bushmen's walking on fire.

The final phase, believed to be a time when participants separate from the spirit, is often a time of bewilderment and confusion as the shakers start to disengage from the ecstatic experience. They may sing or hum, accompanied by gasps, groans, sighs, or shouts. This is when they typically feel breathless and dizzy, while the same kind of random behavior that characterized the preparatory stage takes place again.

How does a shaker know whether he or she is possessed by the Holy Spirit, or by an African deity such as Shango? For the most part, it is the context that determines how things are interpreted. If all members believe that the African deities have been shooed away, then by definition, there can be no such deity present. A few Spiritual Baptists, mainly from Trinidad, don't see any difference between Shango and Holy Spirit inspiration. Bishop Ella Andall, from Trinidad, proposes that the Spiritual Baptists actually blend Christianity and the Orishas (African deities). She doesn't see this as diminishing the strength of either, but as enhancing both. The ceremony does, in fact, resemble the rituals of the Bokono Sage's initiation, and the secret symbols used are similar to the drawings found in Congo.

Rather than using the drums, as in the Vodou or Shango religions, the Spiritual Baptists "use their voices to produce drum sounds that are in seven different forms and rhythms known as 'Doption."[3] One of the greatest gifts you can receive in the spiritual world is what the Spiritual Baptists call 'doption, referring to being adopted by the spirit. Called trumping or groaning in Jamaican Revival, it is a way to cause the shake to become a rhythmically structured movement. Archbishop Randoo calls this guttural sound "the Song of God in man." The 'doption comes up from the pumping stomach and sounds like a drum beating from the chest and a trumpet coming from the throat. This gift is the same as the pump of the Bushman shaman, the pumping up and down of shaking energy within the body. As you pump, the spirit comes through your mouth as a rhythmic expression. This is facilitated by the rhythms of a song. The pulse helps catch the shake and makes it ride a concentrated wave of energy. When you get a strong case of the shakes, you are supposed to learn how to "work it out," "jump spirit," "work penitent," or "work the spirit" and transfer the spiritual power associated with shaking into the 'doption. You still shake, but as with the Bushman shaman's pump, the shake becomes concentrated in the belly and pumped up the chest.

'Doption is the principal way the old-timers would communicate with spirit. Some Spiritual Baptists justify its Christian presence by referring to Romans 8:15 and 22, which refer to the whole of creation groaning and travailing in pain, waiting for the adoption of the spirit.

Speaking of 'doption, Mother Sandy said:

> [I]f you go deep into the spirit you can get the experience of 'doption. It hits you in the belly, tightens you, and pumps your belly up and down. Move when the spirit adopts you. Walk it out. Stomp your feet, swing your arms, and let the sound come out. It will sound like a drum beating inside your chest. 'Doption can show you something. It can bring you a vision or even take you on a spiritual journey.[4]

When the 'doption first brings an extreme tightness in one's belly, it's easy to be concerned. Mother Ralph advises, "When you feel it, don't get scared. Don't hold your belly and sit down. Stand up and let your feet stomp the ground. You must walk it out, stamp it out in a dance for the Lord."

Mother Samuel speaks of strong 'doption as what happens "when the spirit gets into your body." In one of her spiritual journeys, she came to a fork in the road, where

> [a] spirit was standing at the middle of the two roads and I asked where 'doption came from. He pointed to the ground and the Earth

began to shake. He showed me that the stomping of the feet and the shaking of the Earth sent a pumping spiritual energy into the belly. That energy is then pumped up the body, with percussive sounds coming from the mouth. It was so powerful that I went into a top number one 'doption right there.[5]

Like the Bushman shamans with their pumping dance, the Spiritual Baptists know how to harness the shaking and vibratory body energy and use it as a means to go deeper into altered states of consciousness. It can take you deep enough into spirit to travel and experience the spiritual gifts. In general, what we find is that spirited body expression, whether the pumping of the Bushmen and Spiritual Baptists or the whirling and dancing of the Quakers and Shakers, can directly lead to visionary experience. The shaking medicine is sufficient for getting you into the spiritual lands, including spiritual travel, illumination, hearing music, and receiving other gifts, independent of any botanical or sensory-deprivation-induced hallucination.

Typically, the first time you get 'doption is when you are sent to the spiritual land of Zion. Though elder Shakers say 'doption was brought from Africa, in the spiritual lands it is taught in Zion, synonymous with the Holy City of Jerusalem, the most important destination and the holiest place in the spiritual realm. That particular 'doption is often called "number one 'doption," "one-foot 'doption," or "working the pump." It is the strongest and the wildest expression of ecstatic excitement. That it came from Africa is supported by Bell's observation in the 1870s of a dance performed in Grenada by old "Congo negroes" that was identical to the Spiritual Baptists' "number one 'doption." Some scholars think that in a time when slaves were prohibited from making drums and instruments, they made their bodies become the instruments. Bishop Magna Atherly believes that 'doption was brought from Africa and is a kind of "groaning in the spirit." This groaning made the slaves strong and sometimes helped them endure the punishments of slaveholders. "When the slave master met them groaning, they would beat them with a whip, but the power of God was so strong that the whip would fall to the ground."[6] Atherly recalls hearing about a slave master whose son became very sick. When his wife called upon one of the slaves to use his spiritual power, the slave supposedly "went down in a prayer and groaned," and then got up and found a medicinal plant that cured the child. The Bushmen, who are free to make any instrument, also know and express this guttural sound, as do all shakers who allow their mouths to voice the pumping energy within their bodies.

The older Spiritual Baptists tell me that in the old days, there was only number one 'doption. It was all they needed. However, as the pilgrims traveled to other spiritual cities and villages over the years, they learned (in spirit) to modify the sounds and movements to fit the unique qualities of each place. Now there is a 'doption for China, one for India, and one for each of the other places of their spiritual journeys.

Most of today's Spiritual Baptists believe 'doption isn't as strong as it used to be in the old days. In the beginning of their faith, 'doption would bring immediate spiritual sight and transform the person performing it. Now it too easily falls into a more orchestrated way of making music and rhythm. Sometimes the spirit will come on strong, but arguably it is not as strong as it was in the early days.

The Spiritual Baptists' most important ritual is called "mourning" or "taking a spiritual journey," "a pilgrim journey," or "going to the secret room." After having a dream that "calls" the person to mourn, the participant is placed in a small room attached to the back of a praise house. There, a long fast with constant praying takes place, lasting between one and three weeks. Supervised by spiritual elders, the mourners first lament their lives and then pray to be taken into the spiritual world where instruction, knowledge, and spiritual gifts are given. For the Spiritual Baptists, learning in the spiritual world is called "going to school." It is their core experience.

I learned the secrets about mourning on my first visit to the island. One night, I had a dream in which I heard a voice say, "Archbishop Pompey has God's number." I went to my guide that morning and asked about Archbishop Pompey, and found that he lived in the village of Overland, on the northern part of the island. We immediately drove to him, and when I introduced myself and told him my dream, he replied, "Yes, I do have God's number." He told me that I was being called to undergo mourning. In their belief system, God calls you to mourn by sending you a dream of a "pointer," someone who knows how to put you in the spiritual world and point where you should go.

Several days later, I was startled to wake up and find my right arm lifted toward the sky with my body partially lifted up off the bed. I had never experienced such a thing before. It was as if I was being pulled into the spiritual world. This is how the call for mourning can develop. You are called and pulled toward another reality, a place where lessons are taught and spiritual gifts are given.

And so I began my pilgrimage into the spiritual world, as so many Spiritual Baptists had before me. My pointer, Archbishop Cosmore Pompey, now had to vision where I would be sent into the spiritual lands. It might be Africa, Asia, India, inside a mountain, or below the sea. Other cities could be Zion, the Valley of Dry Bones, Israel, Jericho, Sodom, Babylon, the North Pole, the South Pole, Victory, Bethlehem, Jerusalem, the Red Sea, the Sea of Tingling, the Sea of Glass, the Nations of the Sea, Arabia, Egypt, the Sahara, the Indian Sea, the Nations, Jacob's City, heaven, or hell.

I would not be told where I was going to be pointed. That is kept secret from the mourning pilgrim. Instead, Archbishop Pompey would take a piece of chalk and write secret symbols on different bands of colored cotton cloth that would be tied around my head. The colors and symbols stood for different lessons and places in the spiritual world. The "signing of the bands," as it is called, was followed by "sealing" them with drops of candle wax.

When the bands were ready, the community gathered and tightly wrapped them around my head while singing, dancing, and praying over me. I was taken to the mourning room and laid down on the floor. The ritual was to be an enactment of death and resurrection. As I was symbolically buried with flower petals covering me, I was told to review the whole of my life, examining it for shortcomings, wrongdoing, and failure. In this lament, I was to pray for forgiveness and direction for a new life. I was assured that sincerity and perseverance would result in a rebirth and resurrection experience.

As I went through the painful process of lying on a concrete floor, continuously praying without food and water, I did find myself sinking lower and lower into the "ground of sorrow," so low that I could barely imagine proceeding with my life as I had known and lived it. In a desperate and sincere cry for help, an illumination took place that felt like a transformation and resurrection into a newborn life. Ecstatic energy surged through my body and I began to hear songs being sung. I danced with shaking fervor and sang the songs that had been spiritually delivered.

I had known this experience before when placed on the side of a cliff by an Ojibway medicine man. There I had been instructed to lament my life and pray for a vision in much the same way. The difference was that I was totally alone on the cliff, whereas in St. Vincent I had a pointer by my side and a group of elders who came in every sunrise and sundown to pray, sing, and dance over me. Yet the ordeal of praying and fasting was the same.

On the cliff, I remember a coyote coming near me and singing a song. The excitement of that moment pierced my mind and heart, bringing in a rush of pulsing energy that caused me to sing and dance along with the coyote's music. In that fast, I also woke one morning to see myself covered in a luminous fog. As I stared into it, an eagle flew right up to my face and gave me another spirited occasion that brought forth dance and song. In this way, I learned how the old shamans received their songs and their spiritual ecstatic power. They went somewhere in the quiet, as George Fox and his followers did, where they patiently prayed and pleaded with all their might for spirit to arrive. When it did, it often brought a song and shaking energy that burst into a dance.

Similarly, in the mourning room of St. Vincent, I prayed and fasted for an entry into the world of spirit. It came in a way different from what I had known from the North American cliffside. In a visionary dream, I found myself facing an airport terminal with a gentleman dressed in a pilot's white uniform standing on a high platform in the central building. A voice announced that he was "the chief pilot." As I looked up at him and saw his white pilot's cap, the voice said, "Remember everything he shows you." Surrounding him were many different lines and loops and circles of colored misty light. Each of these loops shot out into the distance as a straight line. I remember seeing brown, red, and blue lights on the right side. As I approached the lights, I suddenly realized that this was some kind of advanced transportation system. I immediately felt directed to one of the lights and found myself traveling at a very fast speed, finally landing in front of a mountain. There I received a spiritual gift and began to learn my lessons from the St. Vincent spiritual world.

After your mourning is over, the pointer brings you out of the tiny room and marches you into the front entrance of the church, where the community is waiting. In this celebrative service, you are asked to "shout"—that is, tell what you learned in the spiritual classroom. They call it a shout because typically the fasting experience fills you with so much spiritual energy that you can't help but shake and shout whenever you start talking about your experiences. I shouted and shook so wildly that several men had to hold on to me.

For the first three days and nights of my mourning, I received no food or water. After that, I was given a small amount of water and crackers each day. In the middle of my fast, I began to get very ill. I was throwing up and worried because I was already quite dehydrated. Archbishop Pompey told me he could take me to a physical doctor or he could pray that I be sent to a spiritual hospital. Too weak to walk, I asked to be sent to the spiritual place. It was inside a spiritual mountain where the spirits told me that I had been given unclean water, which was why I was sick. They suggested a plant medicine to cure me. They also gave me the diagnosis for a medical condition that the archbishop had had for years and another plant medicine for healing him.

When I "came back to myself," as the Spiritual Baptists announce their reentry into the everyday world, I told the archbishop what I was taught. Sure enough, he found out that the water hadn't been boiled and that it had most likely made me sick. When I took the prescribed plant,

I became well within hours. Regarding what I told him about his condition, he said I should keep that a secret and never tell anyone else about it. Five years later, during one of my visits to see him, he announced in a worship service what had happened in the mourning room. He said he had a medical condition that his medical doctors were unable to heal, but that after he took the plant medicine the spirits told me about, his problem went away. Furthermore, the doctors said it had not reappeared over the last five years.

My spiritual traveling didn't stop after I came out of the mourning room. I have traveled in spirit all over the world since that visionary prayer fast. Once I went on a journey where I entered an old bookshop filled with rare books. An old gentleman with white hair was sitting outside the shop next to the door. He greeted me and said, "So you are the one we've been hearing about. Please go in the shop and make yourself comfortable." When I went inside, I noticed many rows of ancient books. An old woman immediately came out of the back room and asked whether I needed some help. I asked for a book written by Swedenborg. She handed me a thin catalog and went to the storeroom to see if they had what I requested. I opened the catalog, and the section I turned to was entitled "Esoteric Christianity." All the books listed had Latin titles.

The old woman returned with Swedenborg's spiritual diary. I tucked it under my arm, paid for it, and left because it was closing time. When I came back to myself, I tried to remember who Swedenborg was. I hadn't read anything about him, as far as I could remember, so I wrote down his name to investigate at a later time. I then went back to sleep and had another dream. This time I dreamed I was at a dining table, and a round loaf of bread floated through the back door and suspended itself right in front of me, at face level.

When I was later able to conduct some library research, I discovered that Swedenborg had been a Swedish mystic who began having visions at about the age I was when I started mourning. From that point, he wrote his books only in Latin. One of his first spiritual dreams, entered in his diary, was about a loaf of bread that came to him. He interpreted this to mean he was no longer to be reliant upon the teachings or writings of others. Rather, he was to receive spiritual food directly from the world of spirit. Years later, I visited the cottage in Sweden where he had received many of his visions and went on to the Swedenborg Library in London, where I told my story to the attending staff member. He said, "That's interesting. I work here because I once dreamed of one of Swedenborg's books. It started my journey into the mystical teachings. These are the stories others don't hear about."

The full story of my spiritual traveling and mourning may be found in my book *Shakers of St. Vincent*. Suffice it to say that I traveled to several places and learned numerous things about the spirit. Note that the Spiritual Baptists regard the word *spirit* as referring to three things: the Holy Spirit of God, one's spiritual self, and the spiritual universe. The Spiritual Baptists are well versed in these travels. The archbishop had mourned over twenty times and had been around the world in spirit, as well as deep into the bottom of the spiritual ocean. One of the gifts he and other Spiritual Baptists receive is a role, or a spiritual job to perform for the community. These jobs include being a pointer, bishop, teacher, shepherd, captain, diver, doctor, healer, hunter, inspector, messenger, spiritual mother, prover, watchman, and warrior, among others. Each job is a spiritual role that is taught and learned in the spirit world.

When you go into the spiritual lands, you may enter a classroom where all kinds of things are taught, such as hunting, diving, doctoring, sewing, and baking. Most importantly, you will be taught a song, usually associated with a particular spiritual place. You may also be taught a dance or be given a spiritual gift similar to the ones received by the New England Shakers when they were given spiritual crowns, symbols, bells, staffs, and robes.

In the spirit world, you can receive a job, a name, a number, a color, a robe, or a song, to name a few of the spiritual gifts. You may even receive a spiritual guide who will help you in your work. Mother Brown recalled meeting the angel Gabriel, who blew his horn and showed how she was to build a small mourning place behind her house. Over the years, people dreamed of her, even if they hadn't ever heard her name, and in their dreams they were shown how to get to her house. She would then point them into the spirit world, as Archbishop Pompey had done with me. In this way, the tradition remains alive.

You can be taught to heal. Mother Haynes went to a spiritual hospital and learned how to use peppermint to heal ailments. She was also given a spiritual syringe that she uses to doctor others. In the world of spirit, you can be sent to medical schools, classrooms, and ceremonial settings. You can climb mountains, sink to the bottom of the sea, fly in outer space, crawl down ditches, or pass through underground tunnels. Anyone can teach you, including a biblical character, an ancestor, a plant, or an animal. Even an insect can give you a spiritual gift. Like those in the vision fasts of Native Americans, teachers of the Spiritual Baptists come in all sizes and shapes.

The spiritual lands may present you with a color. Africa is usually green while China is yellow (but others may see different colors in their visions). In Africa, you can learn to drum and dance; in China you can learn to use a sword and become a spiritual warrior.

A spiritual journey can tell you things about yourself or about others. Mother Olliveirre traveled to a garden and looked down at the ground, seeing a clear stream. In its reflection, she observed her belly growing larger. That's how she learned she was pregnant. On another spiritual trip, she walked along the ocean beach and discovered a man with hair covering his whole face, from his eyelids down. He gave her a musical instrument, a spiritual horn that was buried in the sand.

In my own journey, I watched a giant gift box wrapped in red ribbon slide down a great mountain, slaying everyone who didn't get out of its way. The gift inside was the power of the Holy Spirit, the shaking energy that can slay people in the spirit. In another journey, I went to Africa and received a drum. There were some places I traveled, like the Sea of Glass, that I had never heard about until I went there in the spirit.

One of the roles I was given was "spiritual captain," whose purpose is to first get the spirit into oneself and then gather others in the spirit. The captain gathers the people and places them on a spiritual ship in which they travel together. Moving them toward specific destinations, the group goes into the same 'doption and moves in sync with each other. In these experiences, people will frequently travel to the same places and have the same experiences. They will see each other in the spiritual world. It is a group possession, a shared spiritual journey into the invisible worlds.

Every mourner waits to receive a light that enables him or her to travel in the darkness. The light is the most important thing you can see. Spiritual Baptists keep mourning hopefully until they see the sacred light. Mother Superior Sandy taught me that "not every child sees the world of spirit. It depends on the pureness of your heart. . . . If you are blessed you see the lights." The light may be a line, loop, or path of luminosity that takes you somewhere. Or it may be a fog of light, a shining in the distance, or an illumination of the entire room. Prayer from sincere and soulful expression brings on the light, and the light carries you into the spiritual experiences.

"Sometimes people see spiritual telephone lines or power lines on their journeys" and "some of these carry the spiritual power," according to Mother Sandy. As Mother Ralph described it, "These lines are like telephone lines. Sometimes you get a spiritual phone that enables you to use the lines. If you have a phone, and you get a spiritual number, you can dial it and go to another world. You can even dial God." When I dreamed of the archbishop having God's number, what I eventually discovered was that he had received a vision that gave him a phone number of God. When he was in the spirit, in 'doption, he could then imagine dialing that number, and his communication would be sent along one of the spiritual phone lines. That's one of the gifts a St. Vincent Shaker can receive. Mother Ralph says, "As you get strong in the spirit and are able to go deep into number one 'doption, it becomes possible to see the lines in a clear way. If you see the lines you can move toward them and travel, or you can pray for a phone, then wait for your number. You will be able to go anywhere and be able to send other pilgrims on a journey."

Mother Samuel remembered that her first spiritual journey in mourning resulted in the whole mourning room lighting up, even though her eyes were covered with the bands. She traveled to Africa and heard the drums, and found that she could bring forth the rhythms ever since that experience. Years later, when I met her first pointer, Pointer Juke, he told me how strong she was in the spirit and that she learned number one 'doption in her first mourning. As a consequence, every time Mother Samuel talked about strong spiritual matters, she felt a vibration come onto her body. It started as a shivering and then turned into an inner fire that made her jerk and shake. While sitting on her front porch, she once told me, "You can't be sitting down and be cold and tell me you have the Holy Spirit. When you contact Him, you get filled with something that makes you move."

Bishop John defines shaking as "natural communication with God," like "turning on the electricity, bringing forth the current." He describes the "power of God" as "an electric current that comes into your body" and as something "you cannot resist." "It's like lightning." When he feels the Holy Spirit touch him, he is immediately shaken. "I vibrate from my head right down through my body. I feel jolts of electricity. I feel I can throw this power to the people." He believes this gift was part of the everyday life of the early slaves: "During the days of slavery, the only thing the people could do was pray for relief. What they received was direct communication from God."

The initiated Spiritual Baptists know when the shake is coming on them. They first feel a trembling within their body before they begin shaking. That's how the spirit announces itself. For some, "It feels like a breeze passing through you—it makes you feel very light, like you are going to faint, but you don't."[7] When the shaking gets on you, "It really shakes you so you pay no attention to anything except the spirit." As shaking takes over, your body awareness fades away. It makes you feel like you are floating or flying, and when the shaking passes, "you feel relaxed and strong."

A few Spiritual Baptists say that the Holy Spirit shakes them from within and that they feel inner currents rather than overt shaking. What-ever the case, the Spiritual Baptists all recognize that there are spiritual power lines carrying the electricity of God directly to their bodies if they open their hearts to receiving it. Once you get it and continue to cultivate its connection, you find there are times when you lie down that the current spontaneously comes on you. Speaking of this, Mother Samuel said: "Now I simply lie down and close my eyes, usually around midnight, and the whole place lights up. I smile and say, 'Thank you, Jesus,' and I visit Him. Sometimes my head vibrates really fast and my pressure rises."

All spiritual elders deep in the spiritual life know about the lines of light. Some of them, like Mother Samuel, could see when a line was broken. As she described it: "Sometimes the lines have lightbulbs on them and I'll see a burned-out light. I have to go to that line and change the lightbulb." Similarly, some of the elder Bushman shamans speak about repairing the lines of light, fixing them so that others can safely travel along them. They also speak of lines being broken whenever trust has been broken with someone. Furthermore, technological cultures that have little spiritual wisdom, like many of those the anthropologists come from, are described as "folks who break the lines."

Prayer is the key to traveling and to receiving the spiritual gifts, from 'doption to music. The Spiritual Baptists do not believe that simply shaking brings about the desired transformed state. Instead, they see prayer as opening the heart to receive the Holy Spirit's current. When that takes place, anything spiritual can happen. When you go into the mourning ritual, your pointer gives you a secret password or phrase or scripture to use in your prayers. It is like a compass setting that orients you toward spirit. When you are focused in your praying, the Holy Spirit will hear it and come to you, bringing along the energy.

The Spiritual Baptists say that the password "feeds" their spirit. It must be used over and over again to keep the prayers strong. It doesn't matter whether you can read or write, because the mourning room can send you to the places of the Bible. You can travel to Mount Zion, to the Valley of the Bones, or to the Garden of Eden. This is how many Spiritual Baptists learn and believe in the stories of the Bible—by going where they take place. Whenever you go to a place, biblical or elsewhere, any mention of the place in the future will instantly bring back your memory of the emotional excitement and fervor associated with the first time you went there in spirit. Then you start shaking, singing, and dancing. This is how it works. As you travel to the different places and into the various stories of the Bible, the scripture becomes sanctified and vitalized in a new way. It is now a part of your personal experience.

One of the most remarkable Spiritual Baptists I ever met was Pointer Warren, a man so gentle and full of love and praise that you felt as though you needed to grab him and hold him to the Earth, lest he float straight up to the heavens. Pointer Warren also thought that shaking brought forth lines carrying the spiritual electricity. He also saw, as the Bushmen did, "ropes of light hanging from the sky." "Only those on a high spiritual path see those ropes," he claimed. "When you see one, concentrate on it and go toward it. It will take you somewhere."

Pointer Warren taught that 'doption "can give you a vision and even take you on a spiritual journey." He also believed that 'doption is "communication from the Holy Spirit." Its pulling brings on spiritual sight, enabling you to "prophesize, see into others, and even heal them." He too would vibrate when he lay down in bed. His head especially vibrated and his body shivered, bringing on the desire to sing. An ecstasy of joy accompanied his inspired shaking and made him "feel like a cloud." Before he died, he would say, "I'm so happy that sometimes I want to fly away. I want to fly. The spirit is so sweet that it lifts me off the ground."

A shaker named Johnny Jones told me about his first mourning, which was with Pointer Warren. He went on a spiritual journey where he met a woman spirit. She said there was something he should tell her. He replied, "Yes, I will mourn once a year." Johnny didn't know that he had made a serious pledge, and within seconds, Pointer Warren ran into the mourning room, shouting, "Someone just made a pledge. Who is it?" Everyone was quiet, and he asked again until Johnny Jones raised his hand. That's how connected Pointer Warren was to the spiritual world.

In another situation, a group of people from Trinidad came to visit

Pointer Warren. In the middle of their conversation, Pointer Warren suddenly looked at one of the women and said, "When you get back home, get rid of the gold bracelet you are wearing. It belongs to the wife of the man who gave it to you." She didn't know that what he said was the truth until she went home and confronted the man. This kind of story is common for those who frequently shake themselves into the spiritual world. The more one travels that way, the more one's spiritual eyes become aware of unseen things in both worlds.

My pointer, Archbishop Pompey, said that "the deeper you go on this journey, the more the light comes to you." He taught me never to take my eyes off it when it comes. The light has the power to transform and inspire you to enter the most important forms of ecstasy. Like the disciple Peter, as long as you keep your eyes on the Master, you can walk on water. If you take your eyes off the light, you will start to sink. Archbishop Pompey always insists that we must do everything to set our hearts right, turning ourselves away from the things of the world and directing our attention to divine inspiration. Then, and only then, can the most valuable spiritual gifts become available.

For the Spiritual Baptist elders, it wouldn't make any sense to focus on a simple action, like repetitive drumming, hyperventilation, or a specific posture. Yes, it may help trigger an interesting fantasy in a workshop setting, but it is unlikely to inspire a heart that yearns for God's love. Only the latter is able to generate enough spiritual power to bring forth the joyous shaking, the spiritual pumping, the soulful songs that bring forth vocal quaking, and the other spiritual gifts from on high. The archbishop is fond of praying, "In thee, O Lord, do I put my trust. Let me never be confounded."

Spiritual Baptist elders teach that anyone can enter the spiritual lands, even thieves and criminals. Shaking is a democratic expression, available to anyone whose heart is sincerely open to being touched by divine inspiration. When the grace of God's love reaches someone, a true spiritual change takes place and is immediately noticeable to others. This is what the Spiritual Baptists believe. As Archbishop Pompey says, "I can tell that you have become a child of God by how you talk, how you walk, and even by how you smell. A servant of God is seasoned in a special way."

The Spiritual Baptists of St. Vincent are inspired both by the Bible and by John Bunyan's book *The Pilgrim's Progress,* a story illustrating the spiritual journey. Several astute observers have noticed that the Kingston Public Library in St. Vincent actually lists *The Pilgrim's Progress* in its card catalog as a work of nonfiction. The pilgrim's name is Christian, and he meets many trials, temptations, provocations, challenges, and much suffering along the way. At the journey's beginning, his wife and children turn against him, but he says, "I'm leaving the city of destruction and I'm going to the celestial city." The Spiritual Baptists' journey of mourning in the low ground of sorrow is like that of Christian's. The Spiritual Baptists must have faith and advance toward the shining light. As they move closer and closer to the spiritual light, their faith deepens, their hearts open wider, and their souls become wiser. The journey seasons and cures the pilgrims, making them people of the light, shaking lighthouses for others.

The world of spirit works this way, and the Spiritual Baptists of St. Vincent practice it and know it as well as anyone else. What makes their religion unique is that their mysteries aren't revealed to a chosen few. Most of its practitioners have mourned, entered the spiritual lands, and become initiated into the ecstatic mysteries. Their mystery schools are many and never-ending.

What we learn from all shakers, from the Kalahari to New England, from the Pacific Northwest, to the Caribbean, is the high value placed upon spiritual songs. The receiving of a song is probably the most important spiritual gift a shaker (and a shaman) can receive. The St. Vincent shakers call their songs "ships," "roads," and "keys." Similarly, the Bushmen refer to their n|om songs as "ropes" or "threads" along which they may spiritually travel. In St. Vincent, the shakers believe the songs arise from the ground and start the 'doption. Songs are the way you get into the spiritual world. They are passports, tickets, and admissions to the spiritual lands. The titles of some of the songs mention places like Zion, Canaan, the Valley, and Beulahland. Each spiritual land has a song, and everyone who has successfully mourned has received music for traveling.

One of the keys to understanding shaking medicine is found in the music and rhythms that inspire it. Consider that ecstatic experience and heightened arousal don't lend themselves to voicing a calm speech. The excited body wants to shout and sing. When the excitement is channeled through a deep feeling of spiritual love, the heart cries out to sing. As a Spiritual Baptist elder once said to me, "God doesn't talk. He only sings, because He communicates through the heart." Song is the best carrier of the spirited emotions of love and joy, while the vibrancy of music is transmitted through its rhythms.

I would argue that ecstatic singing is a more direct passage to transformational experience than is hyperventilation, posture, or hypnotic entrainment. Stand under the stars and sing wildly at the top of your lungs, doing so over and over again. Throw all the feeling you have into the song. Allow the tremors of your voice to shake your whole body. In a matter of time, the sky will open and you will step inside a vision. It should be no surprise that shamans have been called the "song catchers," those whose hearts are opened to receive a song delivered by messengers of love.

The Bushmen believe this and feel that their songs hold the n|om, the energy that shakes them. The St. Vincent Spiritual Baptists also know that music and rhythm are the keys. The captain of the Spiritual Baptists must sing the songs and voice the sounds that enable everyone to join together and enter a spiritual land. Here the song is both the line and direction they are going, the ship that carries them, and the key to opening the door to the spiritual land. Each song has a kind of shake and movement or dance associated with it, and these movements, too, are learned in the spiritual classrooms. Similarly, the Bushmen learn their dances and movements in a place they also call the "classroom" in the spiritual sky. For shakers, the most important lessons are taught in spirit.

In the spirit world, anything encountered can give you a song. A tree, a stone, a mango, an unseen voice, or another person's spirit can bring a song. When you receive the song, your body jolts and shakes. The ecstatic joy of getting the music is so overwhelming that it is impossible not to shake. From that moment on, whenever you hear the song in public, it will make you shake.

The sounds of 'doption play an additional purpose—they sonically suggest motion, and under a heightened state of synesthesia, the songs may be seen as lines, light, and images of places. As with the Bushman shamans, what is felt and heard is also experienced as sight and even as smell. (Recall Archbishop Pompey saying he can smell the scent of a true Spiritual Baptist.)

The Spiritual Baptists of St. Vincent teach us how deep faith combined with an open heart brings forth songs of passion. These songs, when sung whole-heartedly, elicit a shaking body that can start up 'doption, the classic vigorous body pumping of the ecstatic shaman. In this heightened state, a wide range of altered states of consciousness are available, particularly synesthesia, with its combinations of sensory experience (seeing sound and hearing sight). The Spiritual Baptist switches on these ecstatic experiences not by trick or simple action, but rather by submission to a Higher Being that pours forth a great love into the recipient. Like the Christian mystics of old, the Christian shamans of St. Vincent aim for a divine love and allow it to tremble throughout their bodies, opening the higher doors of perception.

Similarly, the strongest Bushman shamans say they are reaching for the Sky God's big love, allowing it to take them into the farthest reaches of transformational experience and relatedness. What do the shakers say they are doing in St. Vincent and the Kalahari? Do they simply say they are having some shaking delight? They are most likely to say they are worshipping God, praying with their whole mind, body, and soul. Yet they would not say that their shaking prayer is anything different from their shaking medicine or their shaking joy. In the ecstatic experiences that involve a relationship with the highest being, the greatest good, and the deepest love, we find that religion, medicine, art, and play become one.

7

SINGING DOWN THE SPIRIT

The African American Church

All shaking and ecstatic expression is driven and enhanced by spirited music. Nowhere is this more evident than in the gospel music and rhythms of the African American church. Vibrant music stimulates the awakening of the life force and releases the Holy Spirit (or the coiled spring of anointed kundalini), encouraging the congregation to jump with spirit. I will present historical accounts and my own experiences as an observer and former active member in this tradition. I will detail the ways in which they use rhythm and music to enhance shaking medicine.

The father of gospel music, Thomas A. Dorsey, was formerly the blues entertainer Georgia Tom, and in his lifetime he wrote about three hundred gospel songs. His most famous hymn is "Precious Lord, Take My Hand." He said the song was given to him directly from God in a moment of deep sorrow. While away from home, conducting a revival service in St. Louis in 1932, he waited to hear the news that his young wife had successfully given birth to their first child. Instead, he received a telegram that she had passed away during the delivery of their son. Grief-stricken, he rushed home to Chicago, only to find that his newly born baby had also died.

Overcome and unable to know what to say or do, he went to see a deacon friend. His friend, a man of faith, walked up to him and gave this simple directive: "Just say, 'Precious Lord.'" The moment he heard those words, the song immediately came out of Thomas Dorsey's mouth. He sang the song with its lyrics perfectly formed, as if delivered straight from heaven:

> *Precious Lord, take my hand.*
> *Lead me on, let me stand.*
> *I am tired, I am weak and worn.*
> *Through the storm, through the night,*
> *Lead me on to the light.*
> *Take my hand, precious Lord.*
> *Lead me home.*
> *When my way grows drear,*
> *Precious Lord, linger near—*
> *When my life is almost gone,*
> *Hear my cry, hear my call,*
> *Hold my hand lest I fall—*
> *Take my hand, precious Lord,*
> *Lead me home.*
> *When darkness appears,*
> *And night draws near,*
> *And the day is past and gone,*
> *At the river I stand*
> *Guide my feet, hold my hand*
> *Take my hand, precious Lord.*
> *Lead me home.*

A major gift of the African American church is found in its music. In my opinion, the church has nearly perfected the musical and rhythmic forms that release ecstatic body expression. It was a long, difficult journey for gospel music to arrive. When Thomas Dorsey first introduced it, he was kicked out of many African American churches. People called it "the devil's music." When Mahalia Jackson sang one of his songs, "she let loose—sang of and to the Lord with her whole heart, being and body as she'd been accustomed—Halie [Mahalia] got her next big shock. The pastor rose in wrath. 'Blasphemous! Get that twisting and that jazz out of this church!'"[1]

What Thomas Dorsey did was put the blues into the church. The bluesmen had always been the evangelists of soul music, quoting the Bible while drinking whiskey and chasing other passions. When the spirit of the blues came into the church, it set a fire no preacher could put out. By the 1960s and 1970s, things reversed: it was the secular musicians who went back to the church and took its energized forms to invigorate their own musical offerings—what became known as rhythm and blues. Wilson Pickett, Sam Cooke, Billy Preston, Dionne Warwick, and Aretha Franklin, to mention a few names, put the church sound into the world as Dorsey had once put the worldly sound into the church.

What happened to Thomas A. Dorsey is familiar to shamans throughout the world. Desperately yearning and crying for help, feeling incapable of moving on by themselves, they pray for divine intervention, and a song is delivered as a spiritual gift. The history of the ecstatic African American church, whether called sanctified, Baptist, Holiness, or charismatic, among other names, is filled with stories of songs being given to the parishioners in exactly this way.

In the Pentecostal movement that took place at the Asuza Street Gospel Mission in Los Angeles during the early 1900s, there were many reports of songs and music spontaneously arising in the services. Consider this example from Jennie Moore, a young black woman:

> I sang under the power of the Spirit in many languages, the interpretation of both words and music I had never before heard, and in the home where the meeting was held, the Spirit led me to the piano, where I played and sang under inspiration, although I had not learned to play.[2]

Playing a musical instrument in the spirit is not an isolated experience. There are other accounts of this taking place:

While they were praying in regard to going to Africa, the oldest daughter, Bessie, went and sat down to the piano, and soon called to her mother to bring a pencil and paper, that the Lord was giving her a song.[3]

It is interesting to note that Edgar Cayce, the sleeping prophet of Kentucky, once performed in a similar way. As a young man, Cayce lost his voice and could regain it only under hypnosis. To his dismay, his voice went away again when he came out of the trance. Finally, the hypnotist suggested that he find his own cure while under the trance. Not only did he find a cure for himself, he found his career as a psychic. Under a trance state, he could medically diagnose and offer treatment plans to others. What is less known is that the hypnotist tried another experiment with him. He suggested, while Cayce was under a trance, that Cayce go to the parlor and play the piano. Without a single music lesson, Edgar Cayce perfectly played a song on the instrument.

One of the lead vocalists of a well-known African American singing group from Minneapolis told me a similar story. When she was young, she dreamed of a large keyboard in the sky. She saw Jesus in the clouds, and he invited her to skip along the keys while holding a song in her heart. To her surprise, she found that she could play the piano by ear the very next morning.

These stories suggest that there is a way of learning, acquiring a skill, or finding a talent that is brought forth under ecstatic conditions. Whether under the influence of trance, heightened arousal, or spiritual dream, it is possible to "rewire" or transform ourselves to do something we previously were unable to accomplish. This learning by absorption is the classic way shamans learn their art and craft. It takes place in the spiritual classrooms of St. Vincent and was present in the mourning rituals of the early African American church. While in a vision, shamans and pilgrims receive a song that deeply moves their hearts. After the vision, they find that when they sing the song, they know how to perform a spiritual role. The song transports them to the same transformational experience they had in their vision. In that state of heart and mind, they are able to experience and express new ways of being.

The spiritual experience of receiving a song or singing in the spirit was explained by one church member as follows: "You do not use your mind at all. The Lord God uses your vocal organs, and words come out without your having anything to do with it."[4] Stuernagel declared that people also receive divine music that is internally produced:

> The Spirit-filled believer will also be "making melody in the heart." He will have a singing heart. Not everybody can sing with the voice, but everybody can have a whole music-box deep down in the soul. Besides, the vocal song must cease at intervals, but the heavenly heart-song can go on forever. It is the new song of heaven wafted down to Earth which will continue through countless ages.[5]

The internal music Stuernagel talks about is one of the best indications that someone is filled with ecstatic fervor. All the ecstatic shamans and shakers I have met talk about the almost never-ceasing music that plays inside their heads. A particular song may play over and over throughout the day. Or different songs may come forth one right after another. Even one's dreams become filled with singing and music and rhythms. Music is always part of a fully aroused ecstatic practitioner.

Zora Neale Hurston collected this visionary account involving spiritual music from a parishioner from Beaufort, South Carolina:

> I begin to call Jesus too, and that's how I got the Holy Ghost. I wasn't calling Jesus ten minutes before I was gone away in the spirit. I went to the east under beautiful shade trees and the green was like a carpet on the ground. There was a band of people. They all had different musical instruments. . . . I stood outside the ring. The director, he was a man marching time, giving the measures to the music. He just handed me a box (guitar) and didn't stop beating time. I played it. (Ecstasy—"Glory, sweet! Better felt than told! Glory!") I just went to play and went to laughing. Came through in

the holiness, laughing, and shouting in the bed. That was the glorious time of my life. That was the day![6]

I found that whether I was in an Ojibway or Lakota sweat lodge, a Guaraní dance, a Wednesday-night prayer meeting at an African American church, or another sacred gathering, the songs played the same role. They opened hearts and provided a bridge to cross over into the spirit. It is unimaginable to a traditional shaman that anyone could induce a major spiritual experience without a song. More precisely, it's not the song per se that is most important; it's the heartfelt singing of the song, inspired by the remembrance of the emotion that accompanied its first presence in your life, that matters most.

When you are in the spirit and your body is shaking, the songs get empowered in a special way. Your voice gets louder and the vibrations in your body are thrown into the song, making it quake with pulsing energy. This is a kind of spirit singing that helps spiritually awaken others as well as amplifies the spiritual energy of the performer. Moving spiritual energy into the voice and using the voice to project it are well known to shamans and ecstatics. This refers not only to singing music, but also to chanting, praying, grunting, shrieking, and shouting.

A shout at the right moment facilitates the release of the spiritual energy. Shouting in the African American church and other traditions in the Diaspora is a projection of the shaking fervor into your speech, whether you are a minister, deacon, church mother, or parishioner. It sounds like shouting, but there is more to it than a simple shout. The loudness is a consequence of the energized body moving its power into the voice. When it is voiced, it not only sends spiritual current into the congregation, but it continues to increase the strength of the shouter as well. The old preachers think of themselves as sending spiritual electricity into the congregation when they shout.

The Bushman shamans also give voice to loud sounds when they shake. As they pull out the arrows and nails from another person, they hit a climax of effort and let out a loud noise or scream. The sound provides an extra energy boost. The importance of the ecstatic sounds of the shaman and those that are shouted in the African American church or in the Amazon cannot be overestimated. Without the sounds, the shaman or parishioner cannot escalate the strength of the spiritual ecstasy enough for a more significant transformation of consciousness.

Once you first shout, the skill is with you forever. From that time on, the energy in your body will want to go through your voice and make a big sound. This is one of the ways you can tell a big shaman or powerful preacher—by the noise she or he is able to effortlessly and spontaneously produce. As the church elders like to remind us, "Make a joyful noise unto the Lord."

Ecstatic worship is inspired and directed by spirited songs and rhythms. When a song is sung with great passion, its pulse or rhythm is felt more deeply and it awakens a spiritual response. For the Bushmen, the power in the music can be released, and it is held as principally responsible for bringing on the shaking body. This spiritual power was always present in African American history. In the early days of slavery, ring shouts, arguably not that dissimilar from Bushman healing dances with respect to their ecstatic effects, were conducted throughout the South. Adding rhythmic clapping to their music, the dancers would move around in a circle, leading up to a "jerking hitching motion, which agitates the shouter, and soon brings out streams of perspiration."[7] Sometimes referred to as "prancing," the energized movements resembled a horse's gallop. The spiritually aroused dancers would prance around the sanctuary. This form later turned into a march that would come forth under the influence of intensely rhythmic songs. The following account is from the memoirs of Margaret Thorpe, a missionary-teacher in Yorkton, Virginia, who observed one of these ceremonies during 1866:

> When one gets the "power," he usually jumps and shouts, sometimes throwing himself so violently that it will take two or three men to keep him (oftener her) from being hurt; this excitement will last for quite a while, ten or fifteen minutes, then suddenly the poor soul will fall to the floor utterly exhausted and helpless, then near

him a circle will be formed with a man standing in the center who is familiar with some of the remarkable hymns they sing. Those in the circle join in the swinging backward and forward. The motion gradually increases until they seem like a company of maniacs clasping their hands, jumping about, embracing, and crying.[8]

Some scholars, such as John Wesley Work, proposed that the rhythms found in these ceremonies were responsible for the ecstatic body movements, arguing that "rhythm arouses emotion and emotion arouses motion."[9] The cathartic release brought about by this form of "dance therapy" also brought a feeling of liberation. This insight inspired Spencer to write that "freedom-in-religion, which is rhythm-in-religion—or rhythm providing the pulse and the Holy Spirit the impulse—is the empowering aspect that enabled the enslaved to survive."[10]

When the spirited rhythms and music take hold of you, they won't let go. Ask the members of any ecstatic religion, and they will tell you that they are singing praise throughout the day. When I joined New Salem Missionary Baptist Church, in northern Minneapolis, I had the same experience. It seemed like church never ended. I could hear the music and shouting throughout the day and night. It wasn't an irritation or nuisance, but instead a pure expression of joy. It was as if my psyche had no other way to communicate this happiness, so the soundtrack kept playing.

Sometimes I would wake up in the night, hearing a celestial choir with extraordinary instruments playing. This auditory hallucination would continue as long as I felt great joy. If I stopped to ponder where the music was coming from, the sound would fade away, moving from being outside my ears to being inside my head as a distant sound. There were times when a Sunday-morning service would lift me into such ecstatic delight that I would rush home to play some music. I would then sit down at the keyboard and a gospel song would immediately be composed. Some of the songs were later performed by Kim Prevost and Bill Solley, musicians from New Orleans, and recorded on the CD *Precious Is His Love.*

When a song came through me, it became a powerful way to keep spiritually charged. The song I had naturally produced would receive the most internal broadcast time, and whenever I faced a daily challenge, the song would be there to comfort and empower me. Spiritual songs come to people in many different ways and circumstances. They can be inspired by a church service, as mine often were, or from a cry for help. Or the song can come forth through other creative means.

For example, two sisters, Anna and Susan Warner, taught a Sunday school class in their home in West Point, New York. They wrote many books and collaborated on the novel *Say and Seal*, which was a bestseller during their time. It is about a young boy, Johnny Fax, who suffers from a serious disease. Near the end of the story, Johnny asks his Sunday school teacher to sing to him. The teacher subsequently holds him in her arms, reaches into her heart, and a song with these words is spontaneously born: "Jesus loves me, this I know. . . ." That scene gave us the famous hymn, with music quickly composed by William Bradbury, which has been sung by children all over the world.

The importance of song and rhythm is known throughout the shamanic world. When I visited the Guarani Indians in Paraguay, one of their shamans, Ava Tape Miri, told me that a shaman becomes a shaman only when he or she receives a song from the spirits. For the Guarani, being a shaman is all about getting the songs. They enable you to have the power to heal and the inspiration to deliver the word souls. When Ava Tape Miri sings his songs, the women grab their bamboo logs and make rhythms by pounding the ground, while the people dance their sacred prayer-dance, the *jroky-nembo'e*. The songs are undoubtedly the most important resource in their culture.

Songs are the bridges to the spiritual world. My Guarani grandparents taught me their songs and baptized me into their way. I learned that the shaman's songs are the bringing forth of a voice that comes from the deepest part of your heart, and are sung with love and compassion for others. One of the names they gave me translates to "he who receives the songs," because of the way my heart could open and receive their spirit songs.

I found that the shamans of the Amazonian rain forest were spiritually similar to members of the African American church. Being open to the spirit filled your heart and mind with never-ceasing music. In the Amazon, I constantly heard the songs, while awake and while asleep. Yes, the Guarani songs sounded different from the church songs with respect to their melodies, but with respect to how they brought forth ecstatic bliss and heightened soulfulness, they were the same.

Sounds, music, and rhythms in an African American church service pass through several stages. In the beginning of a service, the congregation lays out its suffering and pain. Voiced through anguished prayers and moaning, the beginning of the worship involves a soulful lament, with cries of sorrow and grief. Here the troubles of the previous week and the burdens of heavy hearts are set forth. Parishioners tell one another about their troubles and ask the Lord to take pity on them. Here a preacher might pray:

> *O Lord, we come this morning*
> *Knee-bowed and body-bent*
> *Before thy throne of grace.*
> *Oh Lord—this morning—*
> *Bow our hearts beneath our knees,*
> *And our knees in some lonesome valley.*
> *We come this morning—*
> *Like empty pitchers to a full fountain,*
> *With no merits of our own.*
> *O Lord—open up a window of heaven,*
> *And lean out far over the battlements of glory,*
> *And listen this morning.*[11]

When a congregation is really into it, the whole group will moan or make a chant on top of which a single person's praying voice can be heard. When you pray into this envelope of sound, it feels like the moaning is calling out your suffering and wrapping itself around it. It is one of the most therapeutic experiences I have ever witnessed.

Moaning was an antecedent to the spirituals that appeared on the scene in the early nineteenth century. Ethnomusicologist Willie Collins defines moaning as "a sacred chant of one sentence, repeated two or three times . . . expressed a cappella during prayer, devotion or the preacher's sermon. Moans are melodically embellished with melismas [groups of notes, usually five or six, sung melodically to a single syllable], having a unison and heterophonic tune, and are usually performed in a slow, sustained manner."[12]

"I love the Lord. May His sweet mercy shine over me." This is what one of the deacons might shout out in the beginning. Immediately, the congregation mourns back a line with a moaning melody. Hymns that induce a somber mood are sung and prayers that lament the suffering of the people are spoken. No song is more exemplary than the old spiritual:

> *Nobody knows the trouble I've seen,*
> *Nobody knows my sorrow.*
> *Nobody knows the trouble I've seen,*
> *Glory, Hallelujah!*

Like the Spiritual Baptists of St. Vincent, who aim to clean the space of unwanted spirits and uninvited expression, the beginning stage sets the mood for everyone to focus on the work of the Lord.

Based on secret African initiation rites and possession ceremonies, the African American church service has not only a beginning stage for being somber and expressing melancholy, but another stage for emotional arousal and spirited climax as well. The moanin' takes place in the beginning and then turns into a shoutin'. This is the structure of the original African American church service. It is also the structure for many ecstatic ceremonies throughout the world. Things start out cool and move to hot, begin with sorrow and end in joy, or start slow and get fast.

When the moment is right, the deacons invite the Holy Spirit. Now the rhythmic songs are introduced and the shouting begins. People can then jump with joy, shout, and dance down the aisles. The songs of excitement bring in the spirit. As they sometimes say in the church, "When praises go up, blessings come down." In the 1800s, African Americans were bringing forth the sounds found in Africa, and it scared some white people, who described it as "whining, snuffling, grunting, drawling, repeating, hiccoughing, and other vulgarities."[13] Ever since the early days of the African American church, the spirit has been strong:

> It took some good ones to hold [Aunt Kate] down when she got started. Anytime Uncle Link or any other preacher touched along the path she had traveled she would jump and holler. . . . The old ones in them times walked over benches and boxes with their eyes fixed on heaven. God was in the midst of them.[14]

One way of understanding the movement from lament to celebration is to see it as an enactment of a spiritual drama. First the suffering is brought out and placed in the room. The soul laments its pain. As it is moaned over, prayed for, and sung about, it becomes transformed into an energy that moves from the song to the body. As the suffering is voiced with rhythm and music, it is felt in the body in an emotionally loaded way. The suffering has been blessed by the spiritual music, and its vibrations touch one in a way that pierces the heart. In this time of worship, hearts feel broken and fully opened as the moaning brings on weeping and sorrow.

When the internal suffering is now fully felt in the body, the moment of transformation takes place and the tempo picks up and the words start to celebrate the healing power of the spirit. The body jumps on the rhythm—that is, the spirit—and goes for a ride. This working of the spirit (or riding the spiritual horse or mule) is where pain is alchemically transformed into joy. Making spiritual gold for the heart can't take place unless the raw ore of suffering is present. The pain takes one deep into the low ground of sorrow, like a spring being pushed all the way down. With the announcement of the "good news," sung through the genre of gospel music, the spring is released and the jumping and shouting take place.

The same form appears when the Guarani shamans start with a slow singing of a song, voiced in a melancholy way. Then the bamboo poles beat the ground, starting a rhythm that leads people to move in a circle dance. Similarly, the Bushman songs and dancing merely go through the motions at first, as people gather for the purpose of healing the sick and renewing a sense of well-being for everyone. Then the shamans catch on spiritual fire and the energy is awakened. The songs come alive and the shaking takes off. Even the ringing of the bells in an Indian Shaker service start slow and then build up to a fast tempo as the bodies ride along, starting slow and ending in fast movement.

In his book, *Old Ship of Zion*, Walter Pitts Jr. shows how the movements through the various stages of spiritual performance in the African American worship service not only are guided by the preacher and the choir, but are also influenced by the organist and pianist. The instruments "become involved in a melodic antiphony like that of a congregation echoing the melody of the sermons and prayers as they evolve."[15] The keyboardist's aim is to follow and accompany the preacher and singers, but when he or she becomes in sync with them, it is hard to know who is leading whom. It is probably more accurate to say that the spirit is influencing both of them. Here the influence is reciprocal: The preacher is as inspired by the organist's music as the musician is inspired by the preaching. Similarly, in African ceremonies, the drummers feel like the pulsing bodies are playing the drums and the dancers feel like the drummers are beating and moving their bodies.

In some churches, the arrival of the Holy Spirit was marked by a hissing sound that was contagious, moving from one person to another. It was regarded as the "rushing wind" associated with the Holy Spirit that came on the apostles during the Pentecost. Humming, hissing, groaning, vibrating lips, and wild sounds characterized the spirited services of the African American church. These were arguably residuals of the 'doption, trumping, or spiritual pumping that had come from Africa.

After the lament and the shouting occur, the ceremony enters a final stage. Here the spirit must cool down again before the people can return to their homes. The music slows things down and a final prayer brings their bodies back to a relaxed state. Now the members of the congregation are inspired, exhilarated, and confident in facing the challenges of the forthcoming week.

The African American church, from its earliest beginnings, has always been a "death and resurrection show." In this enactment, they did not shy away from professing their mistakes, crimes, and sins, nor did they avoid facing and accepting their suffering. They used their pain to bury themselves or throw themselves onto the ground, going to their knees in prayer. Lamenting their sorrows and mourning their sins, they desperately cried for God's help. If their call and request were sincere enough, their hearts would be made ready to receive divine grace. In this dramatic play of death and rebirth, they felt the weight of their life slip away as they sensed the possibility of floating upward toward the heavens. There waited the greatest gift of all: the present of God's love, a love so pervasive that it embraced everyone, even one's enemies.

The entry into sorrow and the subsequent march into glory are mediated by the sacred songs. The songs keep the practitioners on the right road and ensure that they get to God's house rather than going down the devil's highway. In this journey, there are more similarities than differences among the shaking traditions. All the shakers are shape-shifters, taking what life gives them, with all its grime and slime, and transforming it into gifts from the heavenly kingdom. In this transformational work, it appears that the deeper one sinks into sorrow, the higher will be one's ascent into glory. If you are too rich and comfortable, it is difficult to coil the spring, making it less likely for a launch into the holy stratosphere. Spiritual work, alchemically requiring the ore of suffering, works best for the meek and poor, for those who suffer. They are the ones who easily enter heaven.

Throughout the history of the African American church, the music and rhythms were as emotionally moving as it gets. The songs of sorrow and the songs of praise worked hand in hand, one leading to the other. This movement is a metaphor for the spiritual road members sought to travel. The highway to heaven is paved with foot-stomping rhythm and heart-inspiring music. It wraps itself around the themes of gospel—forgiveness, redemption, hope, and love—and lifts the people up to the stars that brighten every dark sky.

I have been observing ecstatic expression for over fifty years, from the time I was a child in country revival services to more recent forays into the Amazon and other remote corners of the globe. Nowhere have I seen more ecstatic body expression than in some of the old-fashioned African American churches. I have seen elders who were barely able to walk into the church with their walkers and canes start dancing and running up and down the aisle when the music got hot.

Once, in the Lower Ninth Ward of New Orleans, I watched a woman in her eighties run out of the church, circle the building, and run back in, hustling all the way down to the altar. She then slid into it as if sliding into home plate in a baseball thriller. As one worshipper from the old days explained, "There is a fire on the inside . . . the fire moves on the altar of my heart, and I can't keep still.[16] Another says that it happens because of a "love that wells up in our bosom," and another proclaims that it is "the outward manifestation of an inward joy."

Most of the kundalini energy movements, called *kriyas,* are played out in these spirited services. The tremors, twitches, shaking, automatic movements, unusual postures, and vocalizations pour forth. Rather than resist or fight the movements, a participant allows them to play themselves out. In doing so, the body looks and feels like it is working something out. Like those of the shakers and shamans, the African Americans' spirited performances are valued, seen as evidence of the presence of the Holy Spirit, and leave them feeling both exhilarated and relaxed.

The slaves practiced a religion that included mourning. Their spiritual traveling is practically identical to that of the Spiritual Baptists of St. Vincent:

One night I went to the mourner's bench—I seemed to have the weight of the house on me—and I was in darkness. And whilst I was down on my knees I looked up, and I didn't see no housetop or sky. I just saw the clear heavens, and it looked milkish, and I said,

"Lord, what is this?" And he said, "It is love." Then a shower of rain came down on the top of my head and went to the toes, and I was just as light as any feather, and I had on a long white robe, and I sailed and went upwards.[17]

The early African Americans, including a slave named Nora, were very familiar with traveling in the spiritual lands. Nora describes her traveling as follows:

A voice said, "Follow me, my little one, and I will show you the marvelous works of God." I got up, it seems, and started traveling. I was not my natural self but a little angel. We went and came to the sea of glass, and it was mingled with fire. . . . I journeyed and came to a green pasture where there were a lot of sheep. . . . A voice spoke to me, and it sounded like a roar of thunder: "Ye are my workmanship and the creation of my hand. I will drive your fears away. Go, and I go with you. You have a deed to your name, and you shall never perish."[18]

Like the Bushmen and the Spiritual Baptists of St. Vincent, the African Americans from the slave days saw the ropes and ladders that took them to heaven: "Once again I saw, as it were, a ladder. It was more like a pole with rungs on it let down from heaven, and it reached from heaven to Earth. I was on the bottom rung, and somebody was on every rung, climbing upward."[19] Back in those times, the worshippers had many of the experiences found in St. Vincent. They went to the "low land of sorrows" to "mourn" and knew about a hand that comes down and makes tactile contact. They saw a fork in the road where the right side is narrow and goes to a green pasture. They traveled to a great city; saw God as a person who directed and taught them; experienced God as a big love that made them love everyone; received a ticket for spiritual travel; gathered the spiritual gifts of cups, books, crowns, swords, and robes; and saw the ladder to heaven. For many of them, the ancestors live in the first heaven and the angels live in second and third heavens.

When worshippers were "struck by God," it felt like lightning or electricity, which often threw them to the ground. They believed that this heavenly bolt or jolt brought on a spiritual death, which was necessary before one could spiritually travel or receive heavenly gifts. While the initial impact of being touched by God could be heavy, they immediately felt light as a feather when it was over.

Like shamans, the early African American worshippers used to fast for a vision. No one could be a preacher unless he or she had gone to a swamp or cemetery and prayed, eventually receiving a vision that was a calling or a holy invitation. As on the island of St. Vincent, the spiritual roles were determined by the spirit, rather than human decision making. The vision fast used to last three days, according to Zora Neale Hurston,[20] and when it came to preaching, preachers had to be called three times. After that, the spirit "whips them from head to toe" until they surrender to the calling. "The vision seeks the man" and punishment follows if the call is not obeyed.

This was true for my grandfather. When he was a young man, he kept getting called to preach. He would wake up in the middle of the night and tell his wife, "The spirit is calling, but I just don't think I can do it." Then the spirit began to torment him. One night he was so upset that his son (my father) ran into the bedroom, shouting, "What's the matter? Is Daddy all right?" It looked like my grandfather was in great pain. Finally one night, my grandfather simply declared, "I have to do it. There is no choice. I have to become a preacher."

What is it like to be transformed by spirit? Listen to this testimony from an African American who had been a slave:

> Then, like a flash, the power of God struck me. It seemed like something struck me in the top of my head and then went on out through the toes of my feet. I jumped, or rather, fell back against the back of my seat. I lay on the floor of the church. . . . I rose from the floor shouting; a voice on the inside cried, "Mercy! Lord, have mercy!" I ran to an elm tree nearby and tried to put my arms around it. Never had I felt such a love before. It just looked like I

loved everything and everybody. I went to work that day shouting and happy.[21]

Zora Neale Hurston also wrote about a man taking a prayer fast in a cemetery. In his vision, he was placed on an operating table and opened up, while knives were heard clicking inside him. When he got up, he faced some lights burning on the table. The men who were there told him to reach for a light with his right hand. He took one of the lights, and was told that it was his guiding star. He then was given some balls that were placed inside his chest. After he received a gold robe, he put it on and started shouting. Finally, he was given some seeds and told to watch them carefully. Jesus spoke to him: "Those seeds that come up, they died in the heart of the Earth and quickened and came up and brought forth fruit. . . . And a soul that dies and quickens through my spirit, they will live forever."[22]

When parishioners feel the Holy Spirit, it is impossible to explain its rapturous joy to someone who has never been emotionally touched by it. It is incredible to me that most scholars of shamanism haven't spent significant time trying to understand the ecstatic experiences found in the African American church. It is a laboratory for studying the archaic techniques of ecstasy and, once observed, will leave no doubt that ecstasy arises from heightened arousal rather than controlled hypnotic induction. In these churches, the "transformative power of the holy touch, a power felt both physically (the 'feeling' that penetrates from head to foot) and emotionally (the rapturous infusion of joy)"[23] is performed and experienced several times a week in practically every city in the United States.

Getting the spirit is sometimes called an "anointing." It may feel like electricity, a chill, or a burning heat, and may make you feel like you have no weight. There are two ways in which church members distinguish the ecstatic effect of the spirit. The first is when the Holy Ghost is "on" you. This is regarded as an emotional experience of spiritual excitement, but is not taken as a full immersion into the Lord. The second influence of the Holy Ghost is when it is "in" you. Whereas wild emotions and body movements are fleeting (and shallow by comparison), true anointment brings an emotional intensity and clarity that one will never get over. When the spirit is on you, you are simply reacting to it, whereas when the spirit is in you, it causes you to jump, shake, shout, and do things you otherwise wouldn't be able to do. For example, years ago, in a church in Nashville, there was a man who would get so full of the spirit that he would leap from pew to pew over the heads of his fellow worshippers.

This distinction between display and inner transformation holds for all cultures that work to bring forth the shaking medicine. Workshop-derived shaking in a hotel conference room and self-focused emotional release in a church service have little to do with what the shaman and spiritual pilgrim are ultimately seeking. For the latter, a rewiring of one's whole being must take place to receive the most enduring spiritual gifts. Fervent enthusiasm without spiritual seasoning has more to do with the entertainment of the self, whereas the ministrations of the spirit involve authentic soul work.

The problematic relationship between shaking and ecstatic experience caused by self-centered emotion and that brought on by the spirit is discussed in all cultures that value shaking. It bears repeating: When shaking comes from a spiritually changed heart, it feeds transformation; shaking that is born of human cause is trivial entertainment. Elders of the church caution newcomers to the spirit, warning them that it is easy to be fooled into thinking that just because you shook or spoke in tongues, the spirit has come inside you. It may be nothing more than human display, rather than communication of the spirit.

One of the elders of New Salem Baptist Church told me about a country church in which one of its members had the worst singing voice she had ever heard. But because the spirit was in her, whenever she sang in the spirit, "no one could convey God's love better than her voice." Musical perfection has nothing to do with the presence of spirit. The heartfelt vibrations of a song are what feed the soul of an African American church.

If you are attuned only to the rhythms, the breathing, and the postures, it is more likely that you are performing for an audience that includes yourself. This does not lead to a spiritually anointed shake. But if the songs and prayers are sent up, then the spirit is more likely to come down upon you. Then you "shake for the Lord." This is the shaking that is a gift from spirit, rather than a spirited movement for feeling good. I am not saying that sanctified shaking doesn't feel good. It feels so much better than shaking for shaking's sake that words cannot describe the difference.

Elder Richardson summarizes how the spirit works: "He said, 'If you call me, I will answer.' And when He answers you, the vibrations of the Holy Spirit begin to just go out there—you know, like the Earth when it trembles!"[24] For him and other elders of the church, the vibrations are transported by the words of prayer and song when they are voiced from a sincere and humble (selfless) heart.

The holy touch—that is, being moved by the spirit—refers to these "vibrations." The vibrations can move the faithful at any time, with or without rhythmic music or shouting. Just thinking about the Lord can make you tremble. You can tell that someone has the spirit within when you see him or her deeply moved by the reading of the Bible or the simple utterance of a prayer. That person responds to the words as if he or she is being fed the most delicious meal ever prepared. This is evidence that the spirit resides within. In the presence of the holy, whether it is quiet or loud, the holy within will inspire weeping, jumping, shouting, or shaking. On the other hand, if a person shakes and moves only with arousing music and wild rhythms, it is likely a performance of someone trying to impress himself and others with a newfound human power.

For words to be spiritually significant and reach God, whether in praying, preaching, or singing, the spirit must "ride" you. The spirit within your being, like the Bushmen's arrows in their bellies, must vibrate its loving essence into the sounds that are voiced. Otherwise, the words and sounds don't reach the village in the sky. For the anointed shaker, we can see that prayer, preaching, and song are simply vehicles for the spirit to wrap itself around. In other words, they are like Bushman arrows. When sent into the world and into others, they bring forth spiritual results.

It is not uncommon to hear members of the church say that Satan was once a singer in heaven. They point to the Book of Ezekiel, which describes an anointed cherub who was banned from heaven. From this perspective, the devil can take on the looks and sounds of holy preaching, praying, singing, dancing, and shaking. What this implies is that the greatest adversaries to sanctified practitioners are those who mimic the spiritual gifts. They sing and shake to be seen and adulated. They are not "of Him," to use an old religious expression.

The same holds for shaking shamans, whether in the Kalahari or elsewhere. Some turn from love-based shaking to power-based shaking, and try to use their inner power to influence outcomes that benefit themselves. They practice the "dark side" or "left side," or as the Bushmen say, they walk the horizontal red lines rather than climb the vertical ropes of light. However connoted, a distinction is made between the sorcery orientation (for example, Carlos Castaneda and Don Juan's way) that seeks personal power and the healing orientation that seeks caring and sacrifice for others over the flattering of self.

When someone is shaking or preaching or singing for self, the shaking takes on the feel of "show business" in the way it draws attention to the performer. When it is "pure" shouting or shaking, the self is no longer involved. One becomes a vessel for the performance of spirit. "The only artist singing is the Holy Ghost," as one choir director told me. Those among the church who have become mature in matters of the spirit are said to be able to recognize when someone is anointed. As Archbishop Pompey, from St. Vincent, put it, he can see it in how they talk, walk, and even smell. Bushman shamans can also see who carries the n|om arrows and needles. They recognize the strong shamans before they have started to shake. They hear it in their voices, their everyday movements, and for them also, in how they smell.

When a Kalahari shaman meets another shaman, the arrows flow from heart to heart. They make an instant connection that validates who they are. This moment of connection feels like tingling electricity and often results in a shout being released. The same thing happens when two people seasoned in the spirit meet. Their hearts send out vibrations that penetrate the spiritual veil. They know that they have met a sister or brother in the spirit.

The vibrations of the music are transmitted in ways we will never fully understand. Once, before I took one of my trips to be with the Bushmen, I decided to pour some Kalahari sand all around the perimeter of our house. My wife, Mev, was not coming with me this time, but I wanted to feel that the Kalahari was somehow wrapped around her and our home. The sand had been collected from my first dance with the Bushmen, which had taken place more than a decade before. Men and women had danced and sung over that sand, and it was energized by their ecstatic way.

I went off to Africa, and when I finally came out of the bush, a message from Mev was waiting for me. One night while I was out with the Bushmen, she had awakened in the middle of the night, hearing the Bushmen singing outside the bedroom window. She first thought that the neighbors were having a late party and were playing Bushman music. When she realized that that was highly unlikely, she started walking through the house. To her surprise, the music of the Bushman healing dance was everywhere. It lasted for several minutes and then started to fade away. She had no explanation for the experience because she didn't know I had sprinkled the sand from a Kalahari dance around the house. Perhaps the vibrations of the Bushmen's music had been shot from the sand and received by her heart, giving birth to the sounds that hold the Bushmen's vibrant love.

As the old spiritual reminds us, a spiritual life is about having a song:

> *I got a song, you got a song*
> *All God's children got a song*
> *When I get to heaven I'm gonna sing-a my song*
> *I'm gonna sing all over God's heaven!*

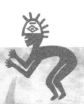

8
SEIKI JUTSU
The Japanese Shaking Medicine

The everyday practice of improvised body movements prescribed by the Japanese tradition of *seiki jutsu* is not very well known by the rest of the world. *Seiki* is the old Japanese word for the universal life force, and the art of working with it involves a non-subtle form of therapeutic touch and body energy work. This almost extinct tradition differs from other Asian energy practices, including kundalini yoga, reiki therapy, and qigong medicine, and singularly follows the wisdom and teaching of one's own body. The work of the great master of seiki jutsu, Ikuko Osumi, Sensei, is almost solely responsible for keeping the tradition alive for the last fifty years. She taught many artists, business leaders, and scientists of Japan to use this spontaneous movement practice to improve their daily performance and the overall quality of their lives. I will describe how she taught me to become her successor and to teach others this efficient, practical, and powerful way to develop a moving and shaking body that heals and optimizes well-being.

In the summer of 1992, I heard about a remarkable woman in Japan named Ikuko Osumi. She was part of the old Japanese family traditions, and her clients included CEOs of major Japanese corporations and some of the leading scientists and artists in their culture. Born as a gifted psychic, she would forecast the weather to fishermen before they went out to sea. Standing on a mountain at dawn, she would wave white and red flags to signal whether it would be a clear day or a stormy one. She also could predict who was going to die and when a baby would be born (as well as its sex), and was well aware of the spirit world.

As a girl, Ikuko Osumi was loved by the villagers and especially by her grandfather Katagiri, who was a very wealthy man. Unfortunately, a tragic tsunami destroyed much of her village, and her grandfather gave away his fortune to help construct a massive breakwater project in Shiogama so that life, property, and fishing boats would be protected in the future. She and her family were thrown into poverty, and it was soon decided that she be sent to an aunt and uncle who would raise her. She was fifteen years old.

Before Ikuko went away, she remembered a time, ten years before, when her family had visited Makiyama Shrine, on top of Maki Mountain. It honored her most revered ancestor, Eizon Hoin, who had been a seventeenth-century Buddhist priest. At the shrine, the Japanese people worshipped him as a *kami* (a divinity) who protects the weak, maintains justice, and guards against fire and difficult childbirth.

Ikuko's family and friends knew about a legendary white snake that lived in the shrine, and they believed it protected them. Its cast-off skin was collected each year and used by her grandmother to make a medicine. On this particular trip, Ikuko was five years old. As she was playing with a ball, it rolled into the shrine. To her surprise, the snake presented itself, raised its head, and began to speak. It said it was very tired and could no longer help the family. "You must do it now," the snake told young Ikuko. She felt its spiritual presence enter her left side and knew it would be with her throughout her life.

As a teenager being sent to her aunt and uncle's house in the western section of Tokyo, she was uncertain about her future. Her father had died of lung disease and her mother returned to her family of origin after her grandfather passed away. Ikuku remembered what the white snake had told her, and she desired to be a doctor. However, to her disappointment, her aunt and uncle didn't send her to medical school. They gave her private lessons in traditional Japanese culture, including the tea ceremony, sewing, calligraphy, and flower arranging. She had promised her father on his deathbed that she would get an education and help heal others. As Ikuko began to believe that she couldn't keep that promise, she became very despondent, feeling as though a "terrible, thick, black cloud" was surrounding her, making her feel disappointed with the direction of her life.

Her uncle took her to many doctors, including both Western and Chinese specialists. She did not improve and fell deeper into despair. Ikuko became curious, however, about a daily practice her aunt was conducting. Every day, her aunt, Mrs. Hayashibe, would go upstairs, dressed in full kimono regalia, and disappear into a small, three-mat room. Ikuko wondered what her aunt did in that small room. Finally, after Ikuko observed this routine for many months, her aunt called her to the room. What Mrs. Hayashibe said changed the course of Ikuko's life.

She explained that every day at three o'clock, she went into the three-mat room and conducted "seiki exercises." Her aunt went on to say, "I can't explain seiki to you, but I believe that seiki is the only thing left to cure you. I am sure I can cure you with it. Are you willing to try?" Without understanding what seiki was, Ikuko Osumi agreed to give it a try. Her aunt then announced that she would "instill" seiki into her the very next afternoon.

When it was time for the instillation, Ikuko was sat on a stool in the "seiki room," as her aunt called the upstairs room. Ikuko Osumi knew her aunt was behind her, but did not know what she was doing. She heard wild noises and commotion. The only other thing she remembered about that afternoon was that she suddenly found herself moving around in a spontaneous way, rocking back and forth without any effort. It was as if some invisible force had entered her, causing her to have automatic motion. She had received seiki.

Her aunt proclaimed to Ikuko that maybe someday she could teach seiki, but then quickly warned, "Under no circumstances are you to teach any kind of seiki therapy. It's too dangerous." Ikuko noticed that her aunt's arms had turned purple and that she had to rest in bed for several days to regain her energy after the installation. Although Ikuko's body knew how to move and rock on its own, she still didn't understand the mysterious force her aunt had given her.

A day or two after receiving seiki, her aunt instructed her how to sit on the seiki stool at least once a day for twenty minutes. She taught her to put the tips of her fingers together, press her closed eyes, and then to "wait and see what takes place." When Ikuku first did this, nothing happened. And then all of a sudden she began moving in a circular fashion and knew instantly that the seiki inside her was alive and well, causing her body to move in a self-propelled way.

Over the days, weeks, and months of her daily practice, her body began to feel stronger and regain its vitality. She eventually found that her hands became like dowsing rods or magnets, drawn to other parts of her body where she would apply therapeutic touch, giving a self-treatment. The force of seiki carried her hands to the places where healing was needed. As she watched her body teach itself how to heal, she realized that she was going to grow up to become a different kind of doctor. She would help her family and others become well through the use of seiki. With seiki, Ikuko Osumi found the purpose of her life.

Seiki not only revealed a "strange, undefinable energy" that permeated her body; it both "initiated a stirring" within her and started an outer movement of her body. It enabled her to cure herself, and it opened the door to spiritual teaching. She found that during her practice, she could "lose contact with the everyday world" and "enter another dimension of the universe." She learned how to travel inside her own body and observe its inner workings. She entered into conversations with nature and learned about the interrelationships between the body and nature, which is the context of natural health. In this spiritual universe, she was taught how to be a great seiki healer and teacher.

During her time with her aunt, she wondered how she could ever give seiki to someone else. As her energy increased, her aunt came to her and announced, "As long as you expect to be taught how to instill seiki into others, rather than finding out for yourself, the more likely it is that you will never succeed. You must master it by yourself." In other words, everything about seiki was natural, non-purposeful, and automatic. As the body moved on its own, the teaching would also spontaneously present itself, effortlessly and naturally, when it was ready. The teaching could not be willed or forced. It would happen in its own way, under its own terms.

Ikuko Osumi realized there was no way to rationally figure out anything about seiki. It didn't help to think about it or wonder what should be done with it. All she needed to understand was that the whole universe was somehow contained within our own bodies, "like a tiny universe of its own." She stopped trying to figure things out, and instead allowed the internal wisdom triggered by seiki to develop on its own.

One day, her cousin came to the house and was very sick. Her aunt asked the cousin, "Do you want to get well?" "Of course I do," he replied. After a pause, the aunt responded, "Then let us instill seiki into you." When Osumi heard the word *us,* she was startled, wondering how she would be able to help her aunt instill seiki. Then, without warning, her aunt said, "Ikuko will instill seiki into you." The confidence in her aunt's voice assured her that it was time for her to give seiki. At that moment, she knew she was ready. She couldn't explain it, but she deeply felt this to be true.

Ikuko Osumi had learned from her daily practice that everything associated with seiki happened on its own and did not require previous instruction. She believed that when it was time to instill it into her cousin, it would simply happen on its own. There was nothing to plan for or think about. She simply had to devote herself to being available for the seiki to work through her. After several days, she led her cousin to the three-mat room without saying a word. She sat him on the stool and stood behind him, as her aunt had done with her. At that moment, the seiki took over. Her hands began moving in the air, doing so with great force. She instantly knew that the essence of transmission was in the hands and fingers. Her hands quickly moved over her cousin's head, looking as if they were "groping toward something invisible to others."

That was when her arms started to periodically bang against the wall. The sound of the impact "sent a strange resonance into my head," and that was when she realized "that this kind of sound was necessary." Spontaneously, she began taking in deep breaths of air and blowing them out with great force as she hit the walls with the palms of her hands. All the noises she made had the effect of triggering vibrations in her body. As she described it, "the room was electrified with sound, vibration, and movement." At the peak of this ecstatic frenzy, with trembling fingers and a shaking body, Ikuko Osumi suddenly felt her hands being dramatically grabbed and pulled to the top of her cousin's head as if a magnet had drawn them there. The force of that movement shocked her. Then something took place that she was not prepared for. Within a second or two, she felt "a bolt of electricity move through my hand into my cousin's head. I knew that this was seiki."

When the bolt came through her, her cousin's head slipped away from her hands and began to move in back-and-forth motions. Ikuku was delirious with excitement. She had instilled seiki for the first time. As her cousin rocked back and forth, she felt "like she was walking on a cloud." Her aunt ran into the room and proclaimed with a big smile, "That, Ikuko, is seiki. You have mastered it at last." Suddenly Ikuko realized that she was bewildered. She had been taught nothing other than confidence in seiki. Later she would come to realize that her aunt had been a great teacher—she had taught her to learn from seiki.

I too once climbed those same stairs, entered the three-mat room, sat on the special bench, and felt the force of seiki come into my body. Months after I first heard about Ikuko Osumi I was contacted by Dr. Kenji Kameguchi, professor of clinical psychology at the University of Tokyo, who asked me to deliver an address at the tenth-anniversary gathering of the Japanese Association of Family Psychology. I accepted the invitation and quickly asked if he could help me locate Ikuko Osumi. I mentioned that one of her patients had been Dr. Takehi Hashimoto, a professor of anatomy at Toho University Medical School, and that he had written the foreword to one of her books.

After trying to find him, Professor Kameguchi wrote that Dr. Hashimoto had recently passed away, and that he had no other way to find out where Osumi lived. Several months passed. The night before I was to depart for Tokyo, I received a fax from my host saying he was delighted to announce that he had found her. She lived very close to the auditorium at Showa Women's University in Setagaya, Tokyo, the place where I was scheduled to give my speech. She had been contacted and was eager to meet me.

I flew to Japan, gave my speech, and was taken to the home of Osumi. She greeted me dressed in a traditional kimono. As she stared straight into my eyes, she told me my entire life history, including information about my grandfather, father, and son. I was so shocked I didn't know whether to shout, cry, throw up, or faint. Then she surprised me further by saying, "You must cancel your trip home and live with me. I will teach you how to make everything you know become one."

I knew I couldn't refuse her invitation. The truth surrounding its delivery and her rock-solid authority could not be ignored. And then I became scared, remembering the stories about others who had tried to learn from her. You had to sacrifice yourself to be her apprentice, or *deishi*. That was the traditional way. The sensei–deishi (master–apprentice) relationship was brutal, and to some Western eyes could be excessive and cruel. I had heard of a professor from Europe who came to Osumi and was instructed to clean her floors for several years. The professor had a nervous breakdown under the teaching relationship.

To my surprise, I was not ordered to clean floors, but was stricken by the brutal truths Osumi would hit me with. She held nothing back, offering criticism, admonishment, and direct advice. She took over my life, yet gave me a place in her home that was equivalent to that of a son. I was watched over and nurtured by her caring supervision. Over time, I was introduced to many of her esteemed patients and went into the homes of some of Japan's national treasures. I watched how she worked with people and how she gave seiki.

Sometimes I would test her. For example, during a weekend trip to Kyoto, I sat down and thought to myself, "I would like some fried chicken. Let's see if she gets that message." On the train ride back to Tokyo, I added another thought: "And let's add some vanilla ice cream to that order." I chuckled to myself and wondered what she would think if she knew what I had done. When I came back to her home, Osumi and her cook were waiting, holding a plate full of fried chicken. Dessert followed with a gigantic bowl of vanilla ice cream.

One of my interpreters, Dr. Burton Foreman, a professor of English at a university in Tokyo, told me a remarkable story concerning what had happened to him with Osumi. He had begun experiencing a kind of paralysis, so he quickly called to tell her about his condition. She told him why this had happened before he could fully explain the situation. Osumi rarely asks her patients what is wrong with them. She says only inexperienced healers need to gather a lot of information. She knows what is wrong. She went on to tell Dr. Foreman the cause of his condition. He had recently dug up a place in his backyard to build a fishpond. While he was digging, he had broken a buried ceramic pot. "The pot you broke was a burial urn. I will give you some salt and sake for you to sprinkle over that area. Each day for a week, you must go to your garden and smile at the place where the urn used to reside." Dr. Foreman's physical problem quickly disappeared.

Dr. Foreman was later given seiki by Osumi on July 4, 1976. He became the first non-Japanese person to receive its transmission. He describes what took place:

What happened was a very strange and wholly unexpected experience for me. On that day I was seated on a stool in a small room. With Osumi were two assistants. They all stood behind me. I waited patiently, although apprehensively. The time had arrived for me to receive seiki. I felt nervous. Quite suddenly and entirely unexpectedly, there arose behind me the most dreadful din I have ever heard in my life. I heard shouting, hissing, and then the sound of pounding. I realized all three of them were hitting the fusuma [sliding doors] with the open palms of their hands.

I experienced another shock when one of the assistants began to breathe into my right ear in an ever-increasing crescendo until he was hissing, blowing out puffs of air, and uttering meaningless bursts of sound, while the other two were shouting at the tops of their lungs, giving forth meaningless yells and shrieks, which produced in total the most God-awful racket one could ever imagine.

I sat there shocked. I shall never forget that moment when, quite suddenly, I felt something come down from above me . . . from the direction of the ceiling, down above my head! Something was entering my head in the back where the hair-whorl is located.

I thought: "My God! This is it!" It was like an electric shock, yet it moved slowly down the back of my neck and into my spinal column. I felt frightened for the first time. Whatever it was, it was inside me and moving down my back. I can say this about it: it was something with a purpose.

But then what followed was even more surprising and unexpected. I saw Osumi and her two disciples appear at my right side and stand, looking at me expectantly. The moving sensation in my body reached the very bottom limits of my spinal cord—the tailbone, and I knew that that was its destination. I was then suddenly thrown forward on my stool in a violent thrust surging up from my tailbone. The upward surge threw me completely off the stool.

The surprise of it staggered me. But one of the disciples shouted at me. "Get back on the stool!" I scrambled back up, but hardly had I sat down again when, just as unexpectedly, I was next drawn back in a swift pull from behind and jerked so far that my legs flew up in the air directly over my head. I can remember the surprise of that so well, because I did not fall over backward off the stool as I most certainly would have under ordinary conditions. Before I could fully digest this very strange situation, I was again pulled forward in a violent thrust from my hips. My legs slammed down on the floor and my face all but banged into them. But—then, again I was pulled backward. My feet were high up in the air again and I was tottering on the edge of the stool. I felt entirely secure in whatever had gripped me in its most powerful, vise-like control. . . .

"Congratulations!" Osumi cried to me, finally. "You have received seiki. It is with you for life. Cherish it."

When I entered her room to receive seiki, like everyone else who had been there before I heard the noises, the banging, the hissing, and the shouting prior to her hands coming down on the crown of my head. I felt my body being rocked and shaken, filled with internal and external vibrations, and recognized that they were the same inner force that I had felt in my own rapture experience in the university chapel several decades before. I realized, in the custody of her vibrating seiki, that I had discovered shaking medicine in many places of the world, from the Kalahari to the Amazon, from African American churches to Tokyo.

When I later showed her a film of the shaking Bushman shamans, she shouted, "Seiki! Seiki!" When I described all my experiences with shaking, she recognized the action of seiki, the mysterious, indescribable force that causes the body to tremble and shake, bringing about healing, well-being, and transformation. When she opened her personal vault and showed me a copy of a historical document written in 1928 by Jozo Ishii, I realized that Japan had been using shaking medicine throughout its history. It supposedly had been a part of the natural regimen of the ancient samurai warriors. Each day, they allowed their bodies to be moved, trembled, and shaken by the universal life force she called seiki. During the first years of the Sowa era, in the second half of the 1920s, there had even been a popular health movement in Japan called "self-improvement life force therapy." Thousands of Japanese people had been moved into health by the natural vibrations of shaking medicine. However, with the many changes that swept through Japan, seiki jutsu all but disappeared from the country and was kept alive, in an underground kind of way, only through the hidden teaching practice of Osumi, Sensei.

What makes seiki jutsu unique is its dedication to natural, automatic expression, rather than adherence to memorized forms. It starts with simple rocking movements that are precipitated by the reception of aroused ecstatic expression. Those simple movements, often involving either circular motions or back-and-forth rocking, are allowed to play themselves out. Sometimes they come to a stop, then change direction, stop again, and continue with numerous variations and possibilities. As the movements are given time to play, an inner fulfillment and revitalization takes place that is first perceived as inner tingling and vibrations.

Most people are familiar with the effortless rocking motion that can take place when you go back and forth in a rocking chair. If you fall into a natural trance in which the rocking feels like it is happening on its own, without any effort on your part, then you have a clear example of an automatic movement. If you now imagine yourself precipitating that same rocking motion while sitting on a stool or bench, you get close to understanding how seiki movement begins. Over time, the simple rocking can become more energetic, with as many motions as there are ways the body is capable of moving. Vibrations, trembling, shaking, and even body pumping like that associated with the Bushman shamans may emerge over time.

Over the years, the natural movements of seiki become your teacher. You never know what movements will come forth until you sit on the stool, press your fingers over your closed eyes, and find out what happens. There will come a time when the hands start going for different parts of your body. They may pat, slap, rub, massage, tremble, stroke, scratch, or shake the body area that attracted them. This is the stage of learning to self-heal. After more practice, your hands start feeling drawn to the bodies of those around you. This is when you begin placing your hands on others with whom you have a trusting relationship. In the Japanese practice of seiki jutsu, family members give seiki to one another in this way, constantly tuning and revitalizing each other with the shaking medicine.

Again, one allows the movements to move themselves. There are no preconceived forms or ideas about how the body should move. As Osumi taught me: "Forget what you have been told about qigong, t'ai chi exercises, or any of the other Asian disciplines. I don't want you to be purposeful about anything. Do not attempt preconceived forms or choreographed sequences of motions with names like 'grasping the bird's tail' or 'wave hands like clouds.' In this approach, which I feel is more natural, I want you to become empty and available. Wait for the seiki to move you."

There are times when others might see you execute a perfect choreography like "wave hands like clouds," but in this case, it happens without aim or purpose. The form spontaneously presents itself and then moves on to another movement. This is how all choreographed practices began in the first place. Someone, in a moment of perfection, was naturally and effortlessly moved by the life force, or seiki, and then afterward, the form was taught to others. In this method of teaching, things get arranged in a backward manner. The form is first demonstrated so the student can memorize and perfect it, and the student hopes that someday, after years of practice, it will manifest itself automatically, without any effort.

Seiki jutsu, on the other hand, cultivates the spontaneous movements and allows the art of improvisational movement to develop in its own way. This practice is regarded as a way to "milk the life force," bringing it into the body and circulating it through pulsing and pumping movements. I have felt the same energized situations in other traditions that honor the shaking medicine. It feels the same with the Bushman shamans and with healers who interact in an ecstatic manner. What is unique about seiki jutsu is that a person sits on a bench to receive the life force. One begins the daily practice while sitting, but with practice, one may be moved to stand and move around the bench. Seiki jutsu reminds us that it is the spontaneous movement, rather than any particular form, that is most important. It teaches us that it doesn't matter whether the shaking is a small vibration or a whole-body convulsion. Its natural and effortless expression is what is most valued.

Not only the fingers, hands, arms, legs, and torso can move, but also the vocal cords. All kinds of sounds will come forth when seiki is being milked and moved. As with the Bushman shamans and the Shakers and Quakers, who, incidentally, also started their ceremonial gatherings while sitting on wooden benches, a wide range of sounds may be emitted. These include hissing sounds, shouts, and an exclamation of "Hai!" or "Vvvoooot!" As with the Bushman shamans, the sound reaches its release and climax as the intensity of the body excitation hits its peak.

Seiki jutsu recognizes that the transmission of seiki, or what we can more generally call shaking medicine, requires openness to reception. A person must be ready to receive it. In the Kalahari, the weekly dances and personal time with a shaman's interactive shaking and touching help prepare the initiate to receive what they call the arrows, the entry of highly charged vibrations. Similarly, Osumi prepares the patient's body to be receptive to future ecstatic interaction. This may take weeks or years depending upon the particular individual. There also must be mutual trust between the receiver and the sender for the seiki or shaking medicine to be transmitted.

Before Osumi gives seiki, she prays that the recipient will be most pleased and happy with the transmission. She then touches the shoulders, head, and lower back, preparing the receiver's body. She believes that the lower part of the back, the sacrum, must be ready to catch and hold the seiki, because this is where it will eventually reside after it enters the head and travels downward. As the body of the recipient is prepared, the sender begins to focus on seiki and nothing but seiki. As the sender feels the presence of seiki beginning to accumulate in the room, the vibrations dance themselves within the body. Ecstatic arousal continues until noises are made and wild arm movements begin. The sender's whole body begins shaking wildly. As this escalates, the seiki is felt becoming heavier and thicker until it comes through the sender's hands onto and into the recipient's head.

As part of my training, Osumi watched me give seiki to others. I found, in the same way that she had with her aunt, that my hands and arms moved automatically as wild sounds were voiced, bringing forth a sense of highly charged energy. When I placed my hands on a person's head, a bolt of energy came through me, transferring an energetic vibration to the person's body. The person would then rock, vibrate, or shake and feel ecstatic bliss. She watched me give seiki to dozens of people, including her own daughter, Masako, who rocked, trembled, shook, and collapsed to the floor in a deep trance. Osumi shouted, "Congratulations! That is strong seiki!"

Osumi flew to my house in the United States and gave seiki to both my wife and my son. She asked me to help give seiki to my son. When I placed my hands over his head next to hers, I could feel a taffy-like substance extending from the ceiling to the crown of his head. I couldn't see it, but I could feel it. With Osumi and her assistant, Taka-fumi Okagima, we grabbed the pulsing, invisible, taffylike seiki, wiped it on Scott's head, and immediately clamped our hands to the crown of his head. He instantly began to rock back and forth as his body was filled with seiki.

At the time of transmission, there is no ego consciousness for the sender and no awareness of a separation between sender and receiver, body and mind, room and universe. There is only seiki, an infinite ocean of seiki, pouring through a channel aimed for the receiver. The seiki actually pours into the body of the recipient, and he automatically receives the exact amount needed to completely fill him up. A carefully tuned sender also experiences the reception of seiki both physically and mentally. It brings everyone together into the room as one mind and one heart. All who are present become a harmonious unity. This is the art of seiki jutsu.

Years after Osumi had given my family seiki and had watched me give seiki to others, she called from Japan, saying she had to see me. She and her entourage flew to the United States and, as usual, she got off the plane in full traditional regalia. That evening, she gathered us and told the story of how the lineage of her tradition is passed on. Whenever any-one is given the responsibility of carrying on seiki jutsu, the priests at the temple that houses the ancestral shrine prepare a special piece of wood with the name of the successor written on it. Her aunt did this for her, and now, she announced, she was doing the same for me. She handed me a rectangular piece of wood with my name in Japanese written on it. It was wrapped with two antique pieces of silk, which were the only possessions she had from her aunt. She said, "You are to teach everyone about this medicine, this way of living with seiki. You are to carry on the tradition."

She handed me a written letter signed by her and cosigned by her daughter, Masako Hayashibe, who served as a witness, giving me the authority to teach the tradition to others. It states:

October 12, 1996

To Whom It May Concern:

I, Ikuko Osumi, acknowledge that I have chosen Bradford Keeney, Ph.D., as one of my successors and that I entrust to him the role of representing and overseeing the teaching of seiki jutsu as well as the transmission of seiki to others. . . .

Sincerely,
Ikuko Osumi

Witness Signature:
Masako Hayashibe

I was deeply honored but shocked to receive the wood, silk cloth, and legal document that made me one of her successors, along with her other successor and immediate associate, Takafumi Okagima, from Tokyo. My mind didn't know how to understand this, but I felt the confidence Osumi had in me, and it was sufficient for me to believe that I had the authority to be a teacher of seiki. She had been like a mother to me in helping nurture both seiki and my confidence in its natural expression. As her aunt had encouraged her to practice seiki, Osumi oversaw my entry into being a master of seiki jutsu.

For a while, I considered calling this practice autokinetics, to emphasize the automatic or spontaneous body movements that bring forth the life force. Anyone can benefit from this simple and effortless daily exercise that brings forth an aroused moving body, provides a natural way of invigorating the mind and body, retunes one's well-being, and prepares one to activate and receive shaking medicine. As a daily practice, it involves the following three steps:

Step one: Initiate the body rhythm. Sit, and start an automatic motion of your body with a natural, spontaneous rhythm.

Step two: Improvise movement. Engage in improvised body expression, ranging from small movements to dancelike as well as non-dancelike postures and gestures, and be open to making impromptu sounds. Be free and unattached to any expected or valued form.

Step three: Enter the shaking zone. Allow this free and spontaneous expression of your body to awaken natural vibrations, trembling, and shaking. This ecstatic zone will bring forth a tuning and recalibration of your whole being.

In the Japanese tradition of seiki jutsu, a wooden seiki bench is seventeen inches high, with a seat measuring sixteen by nine inches. However, it doesn't matter what kind of chair or bench you use as long as you are able to move easily while sitting on it. A flat surface is best, and any soft cushions or upholstery should be avoided. You do not want to sink or fall back into a chair. It should be as benchlike as possible.

As in the seiki jutsu tradition, sit down, take a deep breath, close your eyes, and wait a few seconds. Press the inner corner of each eyeball with the middle and second fingers of each hand. Doing so sends a signal to your autonomic nervous system that you are beginning a session.

At first, your only goal is to jump-start an automatic rocking or swaying movement. The most important thing to remember is that there are no right or wrong forms of movement. What you are aiming for is spontaneous movement, rather than forced movement that fits a purposeful form.

I recognize the "Be spontaneous!" paradox that this situation brings forth. Trying to be spontaneous easily short-circuits or negates spontaneity. One way to avoid this dilemma is to paradoxically attempt "wrong action." This may accidentally trip you into an automatic movement. For example, try moving in any way that you feel is wrong and are convinced will not work. Then try another wrong movement, doing so again and again until you fall into an automatic motion. Typically, in the beginning, this will involve swaying or rocking. But do not aim to rock or sway; that would destroy the spontaneity!

I sometimes recommend that you be completely spastic for a moment, vigorously mobilizing all the parts of your body. Wiggle your toes and fingers, shake your arms and legs, twist your waist, bounce up and down, twist your head from side to side, huff and puff so as to move your chest, and so forth. Do everything that is the opposite of what you might do to relax your body. Arouse your body rather than relaxing it. When you max out or hit a peak with these movements, come to an immediate stop and feel your body start to have a tiny movement on its own. Wait for the natural rhythm and vibration to come forth.

There was a remarkable music teacher in Boston named Madame Chaloff who taught many famous pianists, such as Keith Jarrett and Herbie Hancock. She began with one lesson: how to play one note perfectly and effortlessly. Once you got past that lesson, you had most of what she believed was important about making music—or, I should say, about how music can effortlessly make itself through you. In the beginning lessons, she encouraged her students not to practice longer than five or ten minutes at a time. Any more time would encourage them to drift away from effortless playing. The same lesson applies to seiki jutsu. In the beginning, you should never perform the practice too long, because this would take you into a frame of mind that is too purposeful, serious, effortful, and unnatural. Always perform seiki jutsu with the underlying commitment to having it become as natural as play.

Seiki jutsu teaches us that shaking medicine involves an improvised performance of movement with rhythms, pulses, vibrations, and shaking that revitalize and retune us. To receive shaking medicine, one must first get the natural movements going. We have seen how the Bushmen's dance and its music and rhythms help trigger it. And we have noted how the Quakers sit and wait for the Holy Spirit to touch them. For seiki jutsu, the three-step practice helps trigger the automatic movements.

I have found that certain rhythms are particularly useful for precipitating the automatic motions. You want to avoid repetitive, monotonous rhythms because they too easily entrain and lead you to fall into a relaxed hypnotic state. You want syncopated, unexpected rhythms, like African rhythms, that awaken the body to move. Even more importantly, you want rhythms that unexpectedly change, helping throw you into a natural vibration or shake. I made the CD that is included with this book, *Shaking Medicine: Rhythms for Ecstatic Movement,* while in these ecstatic states. I have used it for many years to help others learn to awaken the shakes and vibrations that bring forth the shaking medicine. In the writing of this book, I had a dream to provide the CD for you. It is one of the most valuable tools I have ever used to help others fall into the vibrations of the shaking medicine.

When you play these rhythms, make the sound as loud as possible. You can use a headset or amplified loudspeakers. As the rhythm begins, try making any movement, particularly if it is experimental and not familiar. Do not necessarily try to dance. Dance too easily brings forth the expectation of recognizable forms. Move in a way that doesn't resemble any dance you know. Look foolish and weird. Try small, medium, and big motions. Consider the first step as an experimental laboratory to wake up the inner spontaneity. The rhythms are designed to arouse, to encourage you to experiment, to be wild, and to trip you to shift without any anticipation that a change is about to happen.

As in the previously outlined steps, the first stage is getting an automatic movement going. Think of it as trying to catch a wave in surfing. Once you catch the wave, ride it for as long as you can. As you are being moved in a natural way, do not reflect on the fact that you're moving naturally. This can throw you out of sync. The same goes for wondering whether you are doing it right. Such reflection takes you away from the experience and out of the flow. Just let it happen. The rhythms are so wild and strong and constantly changing that they will help distract your attention.

As you learn to jump-start automatic motions and then ride them, freely improvising movements in a spontaneous fashion, you will see that your body can, with practice, learn to move this way for five to twenty minutes without any effort. With these movements, your body will fall into a steady vibration, with intermittent shakes and jerks. In the shaking zone, you will feel like you are in an altered state of consciousness. This is when the energy buzzes most strongly inside your body. As Osumi would say, this is when you are "milking seiki." It's as if you pulled up to a spiritual gas station and got filled up with the universal life force. This will play itself out and naturally come to a stop. When it does, press your eyeballs one more time, take a few minutes to relax, and then go on with your activity, refreshed and revitalized.

In the same way that Osumi's aunt said that no words can explain seiki, I must remind you that there is nothing you can understand about seiki that will help you bring it forth. You must experience it. The seiki exercise will help you fall into it. When you wonder whether you have experienced it, you haven't. However, when you finally do feel seiki, you will know it without a doubt. Again, seiki is the same as qi, Holy Spirit, kundalini, n|om, and all the other words that have been invented to point to what feels like a universal life force or spiritual electricity.

The practice of seiki jutsu, like other forms of shaking medicine, prepares and opens you to the truths of the world's spiritual traditions. In the natural movement of the universal life force, you can be lifted into the highest realms of human experience. This is most likely to take place when you think less about your own immediate concerns and enter into more thoughtfulness about others. By becoming emptier of self and allowing the life force, seiki, to surge through, you become more intricately interwoven within the ecology of relationships.

When I first received a full transmission of seiki from Osumi I began to feel as though my breath was inseparable from the breathing of all of life. With each breath, I experienced the whole universe breathing. In my practice of seiki jutsu, I feel my mind and body move with this universal breath. Similarly, each vibration and shake of my body often feels like it is moving with the vibrations and shaking of the earth. This is how the shaking Bushman shamans of the Kalahari experience their shaking medicine. It is a natural medicine delivered from the earth itself.

It's no surprise that two of Osumi's clients, Professor Sako (inventor of the DVD) and Dr. Toshi Doi (one of the inventors of the CD), told me they believed the secret to measuring the life force was to develop a supersensitive microphone capable of detecting its vibrations. Seiki, the universal life force, kundalini, and qi are simply different names for the micro-shaking and pulsing of the body, the vibrations that move life.

Dr. Valerie Hunt, of UCLA, found that the highest vibrations we are capable of making bring us into the highest forms of mystical experience. She recorded the "mind field" frequency patterns of mystics who entered these realms, and found it to be around 200 kilohertz, which was as high as the scientific measuring instruments in her laboratory could record. Compare this frequency with that of normal, grounded consciousness, less than 250 hertz, and that of psychic activity, somewhere above 400 hertz. The highest mystical realms are associated with frequencies that are over a thousand times greater than those associated with other states of consciousness.

I believe that the highest frequencies and vibrations bring forth or are associated with the most transformative experiences we are capable of having. Here the deepest wisdom possible for anyone to encounter is brought directly into our being. Getting to these highest frequencies requires kindness, compassion, and love for others, including one's enemies. It is a realm that Bushman shamans and all serious shakers are familiar with. When you love others, the life force is heated and intensified. As you love in the highest way, the universal life force vibrates you into the supreme mysteries and attunement. We find that the deepest pulses, vibrations, and shaking return us to the greatest gift of all, that of divine love.

It makes sense to refer to the universal life force, seiki, n|om, Holy Spirit, kundalini, and qi as the pulse of God, the divine, or the supreme being. It holds our life and is capable of healing and inspiring it. In other words, God rocks. And God can rock you. The biggest pulse moves us to transform every aspect of our life.

I have seen insurance agents, interior decorators, musicians, schoolteachers, nurses, doctors, engineers, waitresses, clerks, painters, poets, carpenters, and computer programmers, to mention a few, have profound spiritual experiences that were initiated by allowing their bodies to be aroused and spontaneously moved by the energy of life. As I have seen time and time again, no matter what spiritual tradition you belong to, or even if you do not adopt any particular tradition, the natural movements, vibrations, and shaking can carry you into a sacred experience that may completely alter your life.

Practically every mystical practice in the world seems to have discovered the transformational benefits and spiritual contributions of natural movement, vibrating, and shaking. These traditions include not only the ones discussed here, but also the Celtics, Greeks, Tibetans, Hawaiians, Kabbalists, early Gnostics, Freemasons, and Theosophists, to name a few. In contemporary times, work with shaking medicine has taken place among some Western schools of psychotherapy and specialized forms of bodywork and consciousness training, from Wilhelm Reich to rolfing to polarity therapy, among many others.

The leading contemporary philosopher of the body, Don Hanlon Johnson, also underscores how the invention of different body therapies arises from the originator's own spontaneous movements, which too easily become rigidified when they become formalized and taught to others in an authoritative manner. The most promising future for body therapy will be in the direction of returning us to an experience of basic, natural movements that take place effortlessly and spontaneously.

In China, qigong healing involves transmitting or projecting energy into another person's body, helping open any blocked passageways for its circulation. There are between two thousand and four thousand different styles of qigong in China. They typically teach body movements that can be done while lying down, sitting, or standing. The movements aim to help circulate qi. In addition to qigong, there are numerous other Eastern orientations to energy medicine, all working with internally felt vibrations and arousal. These include acupressure, shiatsu, *chi nei tsang, anma, hoshinom, jin shin jyutsu,* Ayurveda, and *t'ai chi chuan,* as well as many schools of kundalini yoga, aikido, and karate. Again, what makes seiki jutsu unique is its commitment to natural improvisation and its movement from freedom to form, rather than from form to freedom.

Seiki jutsu is similar to the Bushman tradition of shaking in an important way. Both have little to say. Unlike the kundalini yoga tradition, with its elaborate texts, techniques, and metaphysics, seiki jutsu and the Bushman tradition avoid complicated discussions and explanations. They are more Zen-like, wanting to avoid the mirages that words create, and instead to encourage the seeker to fall into the experience. As Osumi says, "Simply trust the wisdom of your body."

Osumi taught me that we each are born with a particular mission or purpose. Shaking medicine, whether called seiki or something else, helps us find our destiny. Its truest teaching is to allow life to move us and lead us to becoming what is naturally intended. When we allow life to come to us, we become what we are meant to be. Our modus operandi should not be to make things happen, but rather to allow life to make us happen. To fully *be*, rather than to robotically react, we must be shaken up and set back on the right course. In the rhythms of the shake, we are reset with the pulse of life.

Osumi gave me this advice to pass on to others:

"I have given you a glimpse of seiki, the vital life force," She told me. "You should not live without it. It brings true fulfillment to your life. It is like the tide of the sea that approaches to satisfy and quench the thirst of seashore sand. Thanks to seiki we can maintain our health and embrace each other peacefully, respectfully, and forgivingly. It brings about a generous frame of mind. This generous mind asks that we nurture and prosper with seiki, benefiting ourselves and the universe at the same time. The door to seiki is open to everyone who wishes to enter."

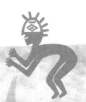

9

COILED WISDOM

Shaking Medicine, Shakti, and Kundalini

In 1932, Carl Jung suggested it would take a thousand years for depth psychology to awaken kundalini, what we are calling shaking medicine, in the West. He and his colleagues assumed that this had to do with the limitations of Western people. I believe that Jung's postulation had more to do with the limitations of depth psychology and psychology in general. Today, we know that Westerners are as capable of awakening the shaking as anyone else in the world. When we walk away from the limitations inherently prescribed by most theories of psychology and psychiatry (based largely on observations of pathology rather than human potential) and accept the more universal truths of the world's great religions, we find ourselves fully equipped to receive the shake.

The Sanskrit word *kundalini* literally means "she who is coiled," and is usually visually represented by a coiled serpent. According to the tantra yoga tradition, kundalini contains a power, energy, or force called *shakti* that lies dormant at the base of the spine, waiting to be awakened and released. *Kundalini-shakti* is literally "serpent power," another way of pointing to the shaking medicine that resides within our bodies. As we have found, it is known by many other names throughout the world.

Gopi Krishna taught Westerners that the extraordinary ecstatic experiences of Christian mystics, yoga adepts, expert shamans, and Sufi masters were essentially the same. He saw them as examples of psycho-physiological transformation brought forth by kundalini. From our perspective, these accomplished ecstatics were seasoned performers of shaking medicine. They were well experienced with the vibrations, jerks, quakes, and shakes that transform one's entire being, bringing untold spiritual gifts along the way.

Tantra yoga proposes that there are seven centers or wheels of spiritual power that line up along the spine. Each *chakra,* or localized vortex of vibrating energy, is represented as a lotus flower with a unique number of petals, which indicates that each center has a unique form of energetic expression. I will compare the chakra model of kundalini movement with the experiences of the Kalahari Bushmen, who, as we have seen, are the most accomplished masters of the shaking medicine.

The four-petaled base chakra is at the anus, and is called the "root-prop center," or *muladhara* chakra. Associated with the earth, the feet, and the sense of smell, its serves to distribute the life force through the whole body. This description relates to the Bushman shamans' belief that stomping the ground helps bring the energy, what they call n|om, through the soles of the feet and up the legs into the rest of the body. They dance in order to help the arrows of n|om come into their feet and legs and then heat up the rest of their body. Furthermore, past and present Bushman shamans have used smell to diagnose the physical condition of others. It is regarded as the first base of assessing what needs to be addressed in the ecstatic treatment of sickness.

The second center in ascending order is the six-petaled *swadhisthana* chakra, located in the genital region. Associated with water, it involves our sense of taste, our sexuality, our personality, and the sensitive use of our hands. When the life force first starts to rise, we often feel it empowering our sexuality and erotic capacities. The power can stay here or it can continue to climb. The Bushman healing dance does not typically elicit strong feelings of sexual arousal. Unlike other African dances and healing traditions that overtly use sexual energy as part of their ceremonial interaction, the Bushman dance usually arouses a body energy that triggers shamanic consciousness rather than stimulating genital sexuality.

However, the heightened feelings evoked by the music and dancing bring forth generalized erotic sensitivities and a desire to touch others with one's hands and skin-to-skin contact.

The next center, the ten-petaled *manipura* chakra, is in the navel region and constitutes the world of mind. It is associated with sight and light. Referred to as the chakra of the life force, it is an alternative base or resting place for the energy after one has learned to activate and move it. This chakra is near the area that the Japanese call *hara,* where the life force is believed to gather and rest within the body. Bushman shamans, along with practitioners of the various martial arts disciplines, also believe that their energy rests in this area of the body, ready to be activated at a moment's notice.

The fourth center is located in the heart and is called the heart lotus, or the twelve-petaled *anahata* chakra. Associated with air and the sensation of touch, this is where the phenomena of the world are revealed in the realities of space and time. When activated, it brings forth the feelings that enable a healer to use loving touch to arouse the life force in others. It is popularly said to be the source of "heart energy." The Sanskrit word *anahata* means "unstuck," which is quite interesting when we note that Bushman shamans believe that beginning shamans get stuck in the illusions of power (and the shaking derived from power) and must get unstuck to move toward the shaking inspired by heartful love.

The fifth center, located at the throat, is the sixteen-petaled center of purity called the *vishuddha* chakra. Connected to hearing, the mouth, and skin, it voices the shaman's energized sounds, called *kow-he-dile* by the Bushmen. Ecstatic shamans know that the spiritual power, the shaking medicine, can build up in the heart and be carried up the throat, where it is released with great vibration and shaking power. The heart-to-throat connection brings forth the sacred sounds and music.

The sixth center, called the *ajna* chakra, is located at the forehead between the brows. Here, mental ideas and abstract ideas are experienced. Depicted as a lotus with two petals, it is also commonly known as the location of the "third eye." This is the source of telepathic communication. It inspires a different order of seeing, sensing, and knowing. It is associated with what the Bushman shamans refer to as "getting your second eyes" or your "new eyes." This may also be connected to the Bushman shaman's experience of "feeling the ropes" that provide nonverbal interaction and communication with other people, animals, and plants.

Finally, the seventh center, *sahasrara* chakra, meaning "thousand spokes" or "the lotus of the thousand petals," is located four finger-breadths above the crown of the head. Here all the senses are synchronized, perhaps related to the synesthesia of experienced Bushman shamans. When the energy ascends all the way up from the base of the spine and through the crown, there is an experience of integrating all polarities and dualisms and a synchronization of all colors, resulting in ecstatic luminosity and bliss. The literature of India describes this region as "whiter than the moon" and spectacularly "lustrous." It is what Inuit shamans called *quaumaneq*, meaning "lightning" or "illumination," and what the Taoist masters call the Golden Flower. As the Bhagavad Gita reminds us, when there is true wisdom, the body emanates light. Accordingly, the Buddha, along with Jesus and numerous Christian mystics, would shine with light when he taught. The most advanced Bushman shamans experience this luminosity in a variety of ways during the dance—for example, as a cloud of light hovering over the dance or white ropes that go to the sky.

Tantra yoga proposes that there are three pathways or ducts, nadis, for the aroused kundalini to travel through. One path straight, like the Bushmen's rope to God, and connects all seven. The other two pathways are helical, one starting at the base side of the straight pathway and the other starting at the right side. The two helical pathways converge at the heart chakra. The right pathway is hypothesized to provide her pathway is believed to cool things down, arguably corr functions of the sympathetic and parasympathetic ner

The goal of tantra yoga and all forms of kund awaken the kundalini and bring it up the middl According to these traditions, if kundalini come channel, painful and harmful side effects can re and the Spiritual Baptists of St. Vincent refer to lines, threads, ropes, stairs, and roads that their spirit travels on. However, these paths aren't imagined to be inside the body, but rather are seen in visionary states as actual highways for spiritual travel. They also hold that there are good roads (or ropes) as well as bad roads that lead to harmful influences and outcomes. Horizontal pathways for some Bushmen may be either good or bad, depending upon whether they are associated with life (green horizontal lines) or with fire and death (red horizontal lines).

After years of instruction and yoga practice, a master yogi's kundalini may start to climb. When it first comes out of the crown, the experience typ-ically lasts for only a few seconds. The ultimate aim is to keep bringing the kundalini up until it resides in the crown center. As the yogi works toward attainment, he makes every effort to not let the kundalini descend the heart. Aroused kundalini that resides in the first three chakras to ego inflation, rampant sexual desire, and an over-emphasis on manipulation rather than love and compassion.

Bushman shamans aim to see the ropes to God and climb They know that they must go past the illusions of power, them to unwisely believe they are impervious to being an enemy, or a hungry lion. The goal of the shaman is to allow love to bring on the shaking medicine and the ated with this empowered way of being.

associated with kundalini match what we have tatic shaking traditions. Although each culture or what it is that moves within the body, each a vibrating and shaking body. From the Sanskrit literature suggests that the ris-"restrictions," or "constrictions" that w. When it encounters a constriction, ense flow of water through a small hip about violently, whereas the be noticeable."

man must be a hollow tube n or her. The teaching is identical. When the pathway is obstructed or dirty, the life force or spirit will cause us to whip around as it cleans and burns away the imperfections. This is not a bad thing. It is a necessary cleansing action. No one can walk around every day with a hollow tube, because we are human. We become filled with many contradictions and existential dualities that clog our ability to see the light and confound our inner wisdom. We must be frequently shaken to continually reopen the pathways for healing, invigoration, transformation, and illumination.

Bushman shamans are well aware of the need to shake in order to clean the dirty arrows that hold the n|om, or life force. The shaking heats up the arrows in order to clean and reenergize them. Shamans clean and empower their own arrows as well as remove, clean, and replace other people's dirty arrows. This is one of the definitions of Bushman healing.

What happens to Bushman shamans can teach us more about the specific way in which the life force, n|om, or kundalini brings forth transformational experience. In the healing dance, the shamans shake wildly, often doing so throughout the night. But after an intense period of wild shaking and jerking, the shaking gives way to a high-frequency vibration, usually felt in the head. At this time, the higher spiritual gifts come to the shaman, and he or she is able to acquire the so-called second eyes, transform into heightened states of consciousness, and perform as a powerful shaman.

After the high frequency subsides, the shaman may move to help other people, feel their pain, absorb their disease, and start to shake again, doing so until the inner vessel is clean and hollow. Then the high-frequency vibrations come on the shaman once again. This cycle repeats itself throughout the night: getting the energy aroused, shaking wildly, then vibrating at a high frequency. This ecstatic ride is the energetic journey of the shaman.

Ecstatic shamans, including those from the Kalahari, are arguably no different from the enlightened yogis of India. Gopi Krishna's description of what he calls a "kundalini rising" could also be the words of a Bushman shaman describing the inner arousal and movement of n|om:

I invariably perceived a luminous glow within and outside my head in a state of constant vibration, as if a jet of an extremely subtle and brilliant substance rising through the spine spread itself out in the cranium, filling and surrounding it with an indescribable radiance. . . .

I distinctly felt an incomparably blissful sensation in all my nerves moving from the tips of fingers and toes and other parts of the trunk and limbs towards the spine, where, concentrated and intensified, it mounted upwards with a still more exquisitely pleasant feeling to pour into the upper region of the brain a rapturous and exhilarating stream of a rare radiating nerve secretion. In the absence of a more suitable appellation, I call it "nectar."[1]

The Taoists refer to this "nectar" as the "Elixir of Immortality," and it is from the highest realm of experience possible for human beings. I have experienced this nectar numerous times in my life, beginning with my own spontaneous kundalini awakening when I was nineteen years old. I was extremely fortunate, for my first awakening brought the energy up my spine and through my crown, bringing forth an extraordinary illumination that presented itself to me as a luminous egg six to eight feet high and approximately six feet in front of me. Within this luminous shape, I witnessed a luminous Jesus, innumerable saints, and holy people. It did not last several seconds or for a few minutes. It lasted throughout the night, what must have been at least seven hours. From that moment, the energy resided in my crown and could precipitate trembling and luminosity with any intensely felt moment of devotion or inspiration.

Since that originating experience, there have been numerous times when I have lain down and felt the high-frequency vibrations in my head give way to what feels like an inner spilling of warm milk. It's as if milk is being poured over the top of my brain. It flows slowly and surely down the rest of my body all the way to the tips of my toes. As it spreads, it brings warmth and tingling energy. I cannot begin to describe the peace, calm, and deep bliss that this experience brings. There is nothing comparable to this ecstatic gift. It is no wonder that the ancients referred to this experience as a magical elixir or sacred nectar.

I once dreamed that Jesus handed me a glass of what at first looked like milk, but upon closer examination was light. When I drank it, again, the warm flow of something internal went throughout my body, bringing me into an intense ecstatic state of bliss. It was one of the most empowering experiences of my life. I have received this elixir in various forms and manners, from receiving it in Kalahari dances to waking up in the middle of the night to find myself encountering a presence that brings the white nectar with it.

Lesua|hun, a woman healer among the Bushmen, had a grandmother who was well known for a special tortoise shell filled with magic liquid. She would supposedly bring it down from the sky during a spirited community dance. I met several elders who remembered drinking from that shell when they were young. It brought the inner flow of warm liquid throughout their bodies and triggered intensified shaking and ecstasy. They believed it was the urine of the god that they were drinking. Only it could hold such a magical power.

I once must have been in a particularly lucid dream, for I experienced myself getting up from bed and walking out of the room, through the back door, and into the backyard. However, I found that our backyard had been transformed into a high mountain that I proceeded to climb along a narrow and steep path. When I got to the top, an old Japanese man sat waiting for me. I recognized him as one of my former teachers from Japan, Professor Kato. He touched me, and the nectar once again entered my body. I live each year with these servings of the kundalini drink, transmissions of seiki, and receptions of the arrows of n|om. It is part of the everyday life of those who live intimately with the shaking medicine.

As I travel throughout the world, I always ask spiritual elders, shamans, and healers whether they are familiar with the vibrations and shaking. If they gleefully announce that it is part of their life, I go on to ask them about the elixir, the nectar that can flow inside their bodies. To my great delight, I have met other people familiar with this nectar. They reside wherever there is a culture that fosters the shaking of bodies as a way to approach the divine. Whether in the Kalahari or the

Caribbean, there is a brotherhood and sisterhood of people who live with this ecstatic tonic, the most distilled form of shaking medicine.

For the last thirty-six years, I have gone to bed at night wondering whether the vibrations or the elixir will come on me. I can never predict when it will happen. It can take place when I am exhausted or fully invigorated, sad or happy, confused or clear. The shaking energy has a mind of its own. I simply make myself available for its flow. Though it may appear that there is nothing one can do to bring it on, this is not quite accurate. If I immerse myself wholeheartedly into devotion for my love for God, the tingling is always present, and this state of being helps bring down the elixir. When it starts to flow, it almost always starts at the top of my crown, feeling like it is on the inside of my head, but there have been a few times when it started in my legs or in other places and then moved outward.

My spiritual path has been that of *bhakti*, extreme devotion to God. When I first felt the lightning-bolt impact of God's divine shaking love, it pierced my heart like an arrow. The gift of bhakti is the most wonderful gift of them all. With it, there is no need for prayer, meditation, Yoga, or anything. It is a straight path to salvation and satori. Yet because of my devotion to God, I want, more than anything else, to pray and sing and shout and dance and shake. These actions are not my means to God; they are my celebration of being connected to the presence of divine love.

I understand all holy things as vibrations that affect the heart, our truest organ of mystical perception. Holy words vibrate into all that is, including us. Their power comes from their ability to vibrate our being. When I dreamed of receiving a floating loaf of bread and found that Swedenborg had dreamed the same thing, another dream followed. I was reminded that Jesus arrived in the world in Bethlehem, Hebrew for "house of bread." For me, Jesus is the embodiment of the Word, the "subtlemost, omnipresent vibratory energy that permeates the cosmos and rotates the galaxies and the atoms alike,"[2] including our bodies. We need only to pulse with the sacred vibrations in order to realize their truth and to become them. We need not know anything, but have to be merely an innocent child, without pretense of knowledge, in order to come to the Master.

Patanjali taught that supreme bahkti (devotion to God) can bring forth a spontaneous Samadhi, or cosmic consciousness. This was true for me and it is true for others as well. For me, my devotion was to Jesus, whose name in Hebrew derives from Yehoshua, meaning "breath," "protection," and "peaceful." In the breathing of his name, I join company with the Semites, "the people of the sacred sound in the breath," and utter their mantra: "Jesus." The holy breath and sound may be experienced through other ways and names, and rest assured, as soundings of devotion, they all aim to bring forth the vibrational movements and raise the spirit to reach the crown of light.

When asked what kind of life must be lived to awaken kundalini, Gopi Krishna, in an interview with Tom Kay, answered that the life to be lived is the one proposed by the Sermon on the Mount. This is a life lived simply, purely, with love and compassion, in which you are "not overly clever" or smart, and in which you don't waste the resources of the planet.

As we have developed our intellect, we have become "pygmies" of spiritual growth, to use Gopi Krishna's metaphor. We must join our intellect with an evolved spiritual heart. Yokes among spirit, body, and mind must be made, and they must matter as if our lives depended on their mutually fostered connections. Shaking is one of the ways in which we can mix the various aspects of ourselves, helping bring forth a unified presence.

Buddhism teaches that any perceived duality between body and spirit reveals an existential conflict enacted in the everyday world. It may be voiced in terms of a battle between a man and a woman, a thought and a feeling, or a determined will and a body desire, to mention a few forms. As Don Hanlon Johnson argues, these presupposed divisions of reality "can be transformed from conflicts to paradox" by the art of healing movement in which "a practitioner typically comes to the experiential realization that such dualisms are mind-made illusions."[3]

Jeffrey Maitland, a former professor of philosophy turned body worker, suggests we are easily mixed up by the metaphysical dualism that holds the mind and body to be distinct. It causes us to believe that our "inner self," typically referring to our mind, is different from our "outer self," our body, giving us a confused account of who we are. He argues that it is more accurate to say "I am my body" and "You are your body." Our self, in other words, is none other than our body. With this shift to a non-dualistic realization of ourselves, we can now say that shaking our bodies is truly a way of shaking ourselves or shaking our way of being.

Once we find our body-self, we must proceed with the honesty and courage to face the dark mirage of our reified ego-self. The illusions of ego-self must die, and we must become reborn into our true-body Zen-like mindless self, doing so over and over again "until out of the ashes of human misery a new life can manifest."[4] Alchemists call this transformation the *nigredo,* or "blackening," and St. John of the Cross referred to the ordeal as a "dark night of the soul." We must pull our true body nature apart from our deceptive, illusory ego, doing so in the fires of suffering and conflict. This is the first step toward realizing the philosopher's stone, the Atman, and the Christ consciousness. The sought-after spiritual gold leaves us will-less, selfless, purposeless, and empty. Then, and only then, can the Taoist winds blow and move us with no resistance. This is when we are empty tubes, ready for the life force to surge through, carrying our mission right along with it.

With the death of illusory ego-self, we are able to stop being pulled back and forth in the tugs-of-war that span the existential dualities of our emotional life. In the newborn authentic life, we embrace both sides of the polarities and harness their tension as an energizing contribution to our creativity and everyday vitality. Tantra yoga refers to this embrace of opposites as a sexual union, not as physical intercourse as it is commonly misunderstood, but as a divine play of all imaginable and unimaginable opposites.

When this multifaceted way of being in the world is attained, one "looks upon the entire objective world that is reflected as surging within."[5] The tantric act of consummation takes place when the feminine and masculine are fused within one body. Then one can say, "What need have I of an outer woman (or man)? I have an inner woman (or man) within myself." With this sacred marriage of opposites, the inner workings of kundalini's left and right pathways merge to become a rope that carries one straight into the divine ecstasies.

The Hopi Indians have also known about the invisible energy traversing a subtle body. Frank Waters writes about the Hopi view:

> The living body of man and the living body of the earth were constructed in the same way. Through each ran an axis. Man's axis being the backbone, the vertebral column, which controlled the equilibrium of his movements and his functions. Along this axis were several vibratory centers which echoed the primordial sound of life throughout the universe or sounded a warning if anything went wrong.[6]

The Hopi describe the soft spot on top of the head as the "open door though which [one] received his life and communicated with his Creator." They also located a thought center, heart center, and solar plexus center, the last of which was regarded as the "throne in man of the Creator himself. From it He directed all the functions of man."

The serpent power was also known in other places of the world. It was in Mesopotamia, Egypt, and Ireland. The Irish Book of Kells is filled with symbolic serpents, and the Cross of Muiredach had an image of the "Right Hand of God," in which "two interlacing serpents appear, one heading downward, the other upward, enframing three human heads in ascending series, with a human right hand above, reaching to the center of a crowning, halo-like, ornamented disk."[7]

The vibrations that awaken the symbolic serpent arise within our own bodies. One of the more interesting movement arts was created by Emilie Conrad Da'Oud and is called Continuum. Its goal is to teach people to notice the natural movements their bodies already have going on within, and to evoke more elaborated expression. Da'Oud spent five years studying dance in Haiti and found the Haitian "liquid, organic rhythms" to be naturally transformative. She subsequently began investigating the myriad organic rhythms that our bodies naturally display, including respiratory, circulatory, peristaltic, nervous, lymphatic, and micro-muscular movements. She discovered that she could teach anyone, including a paralyzed person, to feel movements within the body that in turn can trigger new movements, either previously unknown or not believed possible. She now helps groups of people discover and explore unfamiliar movements and shows how they can start other movements that can change lives.

Shaking opens the world of unfamiliar and new movements, and does so with the surprise that the uncommon vibrations soon become recognized as previously forgotten acquaintances. Whether small internal movements or large-scale external movements, the forgotten vibrations and shaking wait to be uncovered and brought back into our life. They may start as a tremor and end up as a full-blown earthquake, shaking up all the possibilities we had either neglected or feared to imagine were possible. With these movements, our greatest hopes are awakened as we witness the surprises a shaking body can display.

Researcher Itzhak Bentov proposed that kundalini experiences are linked to alterations in body rhythms and the surrounding biomagnetic field. Using a ballistocardiogram (a special low-friction table with a sensitive accelerometer to measure body movement), he found that the heart-aorta system can create, through spiritual practices, a standing wave that is reflected in the movement of the body. This rhythm, in turn, entrains other bio-oscillators of the body, including the brain, the cerebral ventricles, and the sensory cortex, which collectively have the capacity to influence the cerebral magnetic field.

This rhythmically coordinated system can bring forth a polarization between each hemisphere of the brain, causing a pulsing magnetic field. In this condition, the head can act as an antenna and both receive and transmit energy into the environment. Bentov's theory enables us to see that the inner pulses, rhythms, vibrations, and shaking of the body are an orchestrated process that, when properly tuned and modulated, brings forth kundalini experiences. From this orientation, shaking is understood as altering the inner rhythms in a way that resonates, reverberates, and tunes in to the higher realms of consciousness.

Whatever scientific theory is proposed, we can rest assured that it will have to address the vibrations, movements, and rhythms of the inner and outer body. When we look at the spiritual side of things, we move toward the metaphysical truth espoused by Yogananda: "God the son is the Christ Consciousness (Brahma or Kutastha Chaitanya) existing within vibratory creation . . . the only doer, the sole causative and activating force that upholds all creation through vibration."[8]

When we are tuned and moved by the greater vibrations, we quake and shake as we behold the great mystery. In these moments of rapture, we instantly find that all our thoughts and theories "have no greater value than straw," as St. Thomas Aquinas said after having a profound mystical experience. After his direct experience of the divine, he no longer pursued any interest in intellectual matters. This is the dilemma of being spiritually awakened. Those who know about these things often do not say anything, particularly with respect to explanation, because of the vast gulf between words and the actual experience. Those who know recognize that they can't say, whereas those who don't know believe they easily can say. And, I must add, some of us feel that we must say anything that encourages anyone to sincerely cultivate a longing for God's mystery.

The detailed texts of tantra yoga are not photographs or mirrors of the mysteries of kundalini. The chakras are hypothetical and illusory notions that, at best, hint at the experiences of the awakened life force. Although the life force sometimes appears to traverse a straight line, passing through a hierarchy of stations, it is also circular as well as non-dimensional and all-dimensional. Our words and theories provide only approximations of partial aspects of occasional experiences. They are not complete representations of a generalized universe of experience. Bushman shamans, free of texts and concern for stabilized explanation, are more like St. Thomas Aquinas after he had his experience of rapture. The Bushman wisdom keepers allow for inconsistencies, contradictions, changes, and never-ending morphing. For them, there is no need for mapping a linear (or dialectical) progression from a base to a crown. It isn't always experienced that way. Sometimes the n|om or kundalini immediately lights up the sky, and at other times it just shakes. It is obedient to only the gods of improvisation and spontaneity, not the metaphysical architecture of a presupposed kundalini tower of ascension.

At the same time, as long as we remember that our maps are not the territory they approximate, they can be useful heuristic devices to serve our conversations and contemplative reflection. We can see how both yogis and Kalahari shamans hear buzzing sounds, shake, see luminosity, and so forth. Kundalini blueprints enable us to see that sometimes these experiences are patterned, that they grow with maturation, and that they differ dependent upon whether one is inspired by power or love. Finally, the maps of kundalini movement rally us to acknowledge and respect the fact that submission to the highest realizations of unity and pervasive presence bring us into the realm of the holy, where the most transformative experiences take place. As we climb Jacob's ladder, the Kalahari rope to God, or the kundalini spine, we leave our words farther and farther behind, and enter into the spaceless-timeless universe of the unseen and unheard, the great void that is the alpha and omega of eternity.

A direct encounter with the *mysterium tremendum* reveals that one should say nothing and do nothing to be ready for the shaking, the vibrations, and the pulse of life that wait to be awakened and to travel their course, carrying us into our intended illumination and destiny. The dramas of kundalini become, once again, another name for "the death and resurrection show" familiar to shamans throughout the world. Entering its transformational process begins when we wait for Godot, confessing that there is "nothing to be done." As Gary Snyder proposed, "Knowing that nothing need be done, is where we begin to move from."[9] Like the Quakers and Shakers of old, we begin by taking a seat and waiting, with well-fed faith, for the spirit to move us.

Holger Kalweit proposes that "the quest of the shamanic student is the quest for the vital force," whether it be called *maxpe, wakan, mana, xupa,* Manitou, *oki, waiyuwen, moya, ngai, nzmbi, megbe, joja, petara, tondi, hasina,* qi, n|om, *ki, ruach, prana, akasha, inuat,* or Holy Spirit. The initiation into becoming a shaman occurs by stopping all that has been taken for granted. This involves a "devaluation of all values, an overturning of the profane world, a peeling away of invertebrate handed-down notions of the world, liberation from everything preconceived."[10]

Like Swedenborg, we must arrive at a place where we are able to say: "I am now for the first time in such a state that I know nothing and all of my preconceived opinions have eluded me, which is the beginning of all learning, that is, one must first become a child again and then receive knowledge infused into one from one's nurse, just as is happening to me now"[11]

When the kundalini is awakened and the shaking turns into a pulse that milks the life force, our heart and whole being are fully awakened. I once felt myself tune in to the heartbeat of the entire world, feeling each beat being the pulse of Earth. At another time, I felt each of my chakras having a heartbeat, as if there were multiple hearts along my spine. However our heart is awakened, it will inevitably release the truth of God's purpose: We are here to love and to celebrate that love with all living creatures. As the prophet Isaiah revealed God's intention:

So shall my word be that goeth forth from my mouth: it shall not return unto me void, but it shall accomplish that which I please, and it shall prosper in the thing whereto I sent it. For ye shall go out with joy, and be led forth with peace: the mountains and the hills shall break forth before you into singing, and all the trees of the filed shall clap their hands. (Isaiah 55: 11–12)

As we shake ourselves with joy, we will reveal the wisdom of our own bodies. As Walt Whitman proposed:

Re-examine all you have been told at school or church or in any book, dismiss whatever insults your own soul, and your very flesh shall be a great poem and have the richest fluency not only in its words, but in the silent lines of its lips and face and between the lashes of your eyes and in every motion and joint of your body.[12]

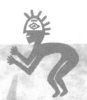

10

THE LIFE FORCE THEATRE

Performances and Testimonies

Over the years, I have literally shaken thousands of people, demonstrating shaking medicine and teaching about it. I have seen how human beings are able to receive shaking into their bodies and lives, experiencing many of the same things written about in this book. What takes place in the Kalahari and the Caribbean, and what used to take place among the early Quakers and Shakers, can happen to anyone, even in today's world. I have witnessed it.

One form of my contemporary shaking work is a transformational and improvisational theater called the Life Force Theatre. It brings people together for an ecstatic ceremony that draws upon the resources of theater and the performing arts as well as the ecstatic energy traditions, including but not limited to what has been called qi activation, kundalini awakening, Bushman ecstatic interaction, and Holy Ghost manifestation. The goal of the theater is to help trigger body vibrations, shaking, and quaking, and to lift people into the highest spiritual and transformational realms. I have performed this work in small and large venues, from the salons of New York City to the Miami Arena. I have seen how the Life Force Theatre can happen in any community, whether it involves two or two thousand people, if they commit themselves to bringing forth the shaking medicine.

Though we are unable to return to the past, and not everyone can travel to the farthest reaches of the globe to find transformational shaking, we cannot afford to ignore the contributions, wisdom, and practices of the shaking cultures. The postmodern shaker respectfully draws upon all sources of wisdom and healing, doing so with the heart of a sincere seeker and the spirit of an innocent child. Avoiding any blind allegiance to a specific directive, the postmodern shaker reaches for the present situation he or she is in and shakes it up, doing so without any overly contrived, self-limited purpose and trusting that a greater mind will shuffle things into a healthier form of enriched complexity. By surrendering to the shake, we become Zen-tantric-shamanic prophets for the polyphonic truths of an uncontrollable wilderness. We shake to enter the vibrations that create, perpetuate, and move life.

Today there is an amplified aesthetic and ethical call for recognizing the importance of multiple views, understandings, and practices. Although some traditionalists fight off outside influences that could change their ways, all cultures and practices are living systems that must constantly change, adapt, and evolve to maintain their continuity. No religion, spiritual practice, or healing way can survive in a vacuum. It requires interaction with other traditions in order to sharpen its own uniqueness and grow.

The expanding horizon of world music provides leadership for how different cultural traditions can support, enhance, and modify one another. Today's global music scene freely takes rhythms and sounds from any and all cultural traditions. African rhythms mix with Broadway tunes, while Cuban rhythms interact with Brazilian songs. Their combinations enhance each tradition and bring new vitality from never-before-heard mixes. I argue that the same should hold for spiritual and healing practices. Respectful engagement and interaction among different healing ways can lead to the enhancement of all ways. Furthermore, shaking medicine can be naturally wed with the diverse styles of world music and the innumerable offerings of the performing arts, and all of them together can be a liberating force in the evolution of the healing arts.

Wherever ecstatic shamans bring down the spirit and enter into a performance of the wild, you have a Life Force Theatre. These performances take place all over the world, from the Amazon to the Kalahari and even to the great urban centers. They constitute opportunities for experiential learning and transformation. They may take place with or without music, special lighting, or stage props. The spirited event can happen indoors or outdoors. The shaking that emerges can be transformative whether it arises from a quiet encounter or explodes with multimedia image and sound. It can begin in quiet anticipation, as the Quakers used to practice, or it can be announced by the fervent drumming of an African village.

I find that a Life Force Theatre is enhanced, amplified, and brought to its fullest glory when spirited music and rhythms are brought into the production. Africa has taken the lead in teaching us how "it don't mean a thing if it ain't got that swing." As I have mentioned before, wild rhythms (like those on the enclosed CD) can facilitate a rhythmic awakening of the shake in your body. Use them when you perform the shake, and use them when you gather people to have a shaking party, a shaking ceremony, a shaking healing, or a shaking happening—that is, a Life Force Theatre.

I have used percussionists, bands, vocalists, improvisational artists who painted the walls during a performance, dancers, you name it. Special lighting, incense, water, stones, sacred objects, comedic interruptions, prayers, nonsense, noises, and so forth are also suitable for this improvisational art. Whoever and whatever shows up to the theater is utilized. It begins with some tinkering—sometimes words, sometimes actions, sometimes both or neither—and waits eagerly until an inspiration triggers the entry of spirited expression. And then off we go, riding the wild currents, letting them rise and fall as they wish, keeping our hands off the control stick while holding on to the spirit and going along for a spirited ride.

Come to the Life Force Theatre for all the reasons you can imagine. The Bushmen don't show up for a shaking dance with an overly serious attitude. If you ask them why they dance and shake, they will say that it makes them feel good, it is entertaining, it is their worship, it doctors them, and it helps the community. All these reasons bring forth the shaking. With this in mind, you can call the shake not only a shaking medicine, but also shaking play, shaking fun, shaking prayer, shaking art, and shaking theater. Don't leave any reason for shaking out of the picture. It's a multifaceted, anarchical experience for a postmodern entry into the wild.

Don't forget to be mindful of the sacred when the shaking starts getting to you. As we've seen, there's more going on than hyperventilation, specialized postures, and sonic driving. This is also holy work, especially when a devoted heart opens itself to the unspeakable and unheard mysteries and makes ready for the epiphanies that can transform a life and empower a community. Bring all your cherished beliefs to your performance, from scriptures to glossolalia, from mystery symbols to mandalas, from songs to shouts, from prayers to mantras. Embed the deepest meanings of your life into your Life Force Theatre. But do so only when you are inspired by the creative impulse, not because you feel you should. Working with the spirit is a delicate matter. It wakes up to the call of spontaneity and divine play, and hides when it encounters the smell of habituated routine, overly driven purpose, and sanctimonious piety.

Of course, there is no way to completely dismiss structure, ritual, and choreography. What we want to strive for is having these forms by our side as we wait for the spirit to call forth what it specifically wants us to perform. For example, there is an established collection of hymns in a sanctified church, and it is assured that some of them will be sung in each gathering that works the spirit. But the selection of the particular songs and how they are performed and sequenced are left to the spontaneity of the occasion.

I have shaken in so many different settings and cultures that it feels natural for me to shake anywhere. I must say that when I am in a particular culture, its spiritual way feels like a complete truth during the moments that I am participating. And then when I am in another cultural setting, it feels as authentic as the one I had been in before. It used to make me very confused if I ever stopped to intellectually ponder which setting or culture or religion was the most enhancing for me. It is the wrong question and cannot be answered, because the particulars of the immediate situation specify what is perfect for the moment.

Shaking medicine, in its fullest form, is a true improvisational art. No rattle, drum, costume, or mojo is needed to get the fullest benefits from the shake. But if those sacred objects are present, utilize them. They will enhance the moment if they belong to the moment. But don't get hung up thinking they have to be there. As there should be no attachment to a particular form of movement, likewise there should be no attachment to any thing. The shaking art requires using whatever the situation brings.

I have found undergraduate classrooms to become as holy as the most sanctified churches. Once I invited a group of students, all between eighteen and twenty-one years old, to believe that they could experience the Kalahari in an old classroom in Santa Fe, New Mexico. They surrendered to that possibility, and we experientially went into the shaking universe of the Bushman shamans. Some of us felt the "ropes," and they pulled us around the room in the same manner that the Bushmen are familiar with. Several students had the most transformational experience of their lives, and for over a month, the campus could not stop talking about what happened. There were no drums, rattles, or holy objects. There were only open-minded people with open hearts ready to be touched by spirited expression with the same degree of sincerity as the early-day Shakers.

I have introduced the shake to Unity church services and other church communities that are typically familiar only with quiet practices. However, they were jumping and bounced by the energy within seconds. It takes no preparation. It just happens when you say yes to it. This yes must come from your deepest unconscious mind, allowing your whole being to be free and available for some shaking and baking.

All Life Force Theatres are jazz. There are standard tunes that help jump-start its movement, but when the spirit of improvisation comes through, the jazz takes off. Shaking is a metaphor for changing, shifting, and jamming. It accepts the music at hand and plays with it, providing embellishment, transitions, and transformations of melody, rhythm, and identity.

It is no accident that there has been a lot of shamanic shaking going on with the masters of the blues, rock and roll, and jazz. Ray Charles, Betty Carter, Jimi Hendrix, Muddy Waters, Charlie Parker, James Brown, Aretha Franklin, and Errol Garner, among many others, have helped keep alive the vibrant pulse of the Life Force Theatre. Now it's time to carry the jazz, blues, and rock farther than the vibrating air and place them directly into the bodies and the interactions of the people who are moved by their influence.

The soulful shaking of a Life Force Theatre heals not only the mind and body, but also the soul. Through this kind of vibration and movement, a tuning of one's whole being takes place. Dr. Robert Fulford was an osteopathic physician whom Dr. Andrew Weil described in his book *Spontaneous Health* as one of the greatest healers he ever met. Dr. Weil wrote in the introduction of one of Fulford's books, "[I]f medicine is to come back in alignment with the great healing traditions and satisfy the needs and desires of those who are sick, it must recover the truths that Bob Fulford expresses."[1] Though Dr. Andrew Weil makes this claim, and begins his own best-selling book with an exaltation of Dr. Fulford's orientation to medicine, he does not proceed to clearly tell his audience or emphasize in his own work what it is that Dr. Fulford believed and practiced.

Dr. Fulford and I knew each other. We had several opportunities to discuss shaking medicine, and he believed it to be the newest and oldest cure on Earth. Throughout his medical career, he seldom prescribed chemical medicines, but instead administered vibrations to his patient's bodies. Famous for curing chronic ear infections in infants, he did it not with antibiotics, but with human touch and movement. He wasn't impressed with the tendency of alternative, complementary, and integrative medicine to over-emphasize the ingestion of alternative tonics, whether vitamins or herbal medicines. He wanted to see medicine follow the trail of the healing vibrations.

When I presented my ideas about shaking medicine to Dr. Fulford, he joyfully embraced them, saying that working with the universal life force, rather than synthetic or natural drugs, is the most promising future of medicine. I showed him how various cultures use shaking medicine, and his response was as follows:

> Dr. Keeney's work marks the beginning of an awakening of the universal life force that is accessible to everyone. I have personally experienced his method of moving the life force in my own body—circulating it up and down my spine, passing it through my fingertips, and feeling it tingling the tips of my toes. It is time for each of us to be acquainted with this energizing force and bring it into our daily life.

Dr. Fulford was talking about two ways that I showed him of bringing the vibrations and shaking into the body. I first showed him the daily practice of seiki jutsu, which anyone can perform. This you are already familiar with. In addition, I demonstrated a particular hands-on way of passing on the shake. It involves my left hand being placed just above the person's heart while my right hand is on the back shoulder behind the heart. I then allow the vibrations to pulse in a spontaneous way. I don't make it happen. It just automatically starts. This is how it works for all experienced shakers and ecstatic shamans. We know how to "step into the vibrations," and anyone holding on to us will also feel them. The vibrations in the left and right hands are usually different, often polyrhythmic and syncopated. They are usually gentle but pronounced, and awaken a high frequency. The vibrations typically spread throughout a person's body, and the effects are immediate and often dramatic.

When I demonstrated this way of shaking to Dr. Fulford, he exclaimed that it was the key to healing that he had spent his whole career trying to find. In a letter, he wrote: "I have found that your technique of starting first, working the left shoulder and heart area, to be very effective in treating. It seems to unlock the rest of the problems." He said further that this way of transmitting a vibration was the highest form of healing he had ever experienced. In the last years of his life, he treated others only with this method.

Dr. Fulford believed that this particular way of administering shakes and vibrations by human touch should be known by the healing community. The most powerful Bushman shamans practice this vibrating encounter, and they recognize it as the strongest form of shaking medicine. It heals, according to Dr. Fulford, through tuning in to the highest frequencies that affect the soul. These frequencies, in turn, recalibrate the mind and body.

I suggest two important ways of becoming familiar with shaking medicine: First of all, everyone can bring vibrations and shaking into his or her life, particularly if fostered by special rhythms and natural practices like seiki jutsu. From my own personal experience, I have found wild, unpredictable rhythms helpful for tinkering with experimental movements that can precipitate spontaneous vibrations. And seiki jutsu is the simplest method available to cultivate natural movements and vibrations.

The second means of receiving shaking medicine involves hands-on interaction with a master of the shaking medicine or the universal life force. I have spent the last sixteen years traveling the world in search of those who have this kind of mastery. There are few "grandmasters" left. It is vitally important that these individuals have opportunities to pass on the shaking to others so that it may spread and proliferate in the world. Part of my responsibility is to help pass the shake to others.

I have worked with numerous masters from around the world, and after thirty-six years of shaking have acquired proficiency at administering it to individuals and groups. I have seen that although there are few grandmasters, there are many people who are ready to help pass the shake into others. They are ready to be activated, so to speak, and then are ready to go. As they foster their talent, they will grow and learn how to use it more effectively. They only need to be encouraged to learn from the shaking medicine—the learning that can't be expressed in words, but accessed only through the experience of shaking.

My shaking takes many different forms, including hand, arm, and leg trembling, varieties of head movements, body swaying, vibrating, oscillating, convulsing, jolts, and jumps. My body's shaking source sometimes comes from the base of my spine. When this is the case, my body typically vibrates in a slow, even rhythm, and I express the choreographed movement of a snakelike form. The emergent patterns are so natural that it seems as if they are being done by an outside source. It requires no bodily effort, and I can sustain such movements for hours.

When the energy comes from my solar plexus, the body vibrations and shaking can be very intense, with fast pulses and rhythms. My body may be shaken either vertically or horizontally, or back and forth across these dimensions. The source of the movements may also come from my hips, where each side vibrates back and forth, shooting pulses of rhythm throughout my body. I am able to choose a spot on my body and have it become a vibrating source for other parts. Or I can take energies, vibrations, and shakes from one part of my body and direct them to another part.

Shaking medicine is different from any spiritual dancing, aerobics, trance dancing, or bodywork I have experienced or witnessed. It is not the ecstatic dancing of Gabrielle Roth or the organized whirling of the Sufis, though it may include automatic movements that are familiar to other orientations. However, here they serve to help bring forth the shaking medicine. In this spirited expression, the shake and the vibration are more important than the dance.

When I shake someone, I often begin by touching him or her in the way I described shaking Dr. Fulford, where my left hand is over the heart and my right hand over the area of the left shoulder blade. Upon immediate contact, I send high frequencies of vibrations into the body with my right and left hands and arms. My left and right hands pulse back and forth, establishing waves of energy through the body between the shoulder and heart areas. My knees may also lock onto the other person's knees and shake at the same time.

If the person seems a bit anxious about the work, I don't begin this quickly. I may touch him or her with light fluttering hand movements that I will occasionally increase and decrease as an introduction to the shaking medicine. As the person becomes more comfortable, I move into deeper and stronger levels of shaking. I don't know how I know how to regulate this process. It simply happens.

For some people, intense work is possible with the first touch. I may work on specific areas or the whole body. I will pull and shake entire limbs, send patterns of waves down spines, do arm and hand dances on backs, vibrate each finger, and move whole bodies into rapid pulses. I also do a lot of shaking work on people's heads, vibrating, pulsing and dancing them. There are times when this work feels like playing the keyboard. It is the same way I open up to receive music and allow my fingers to have a life of their own. The movements are often so quick, ever-changing, and intense that people's minds can't keep up or track them. They are faster than their minds are able to pattern and interpret.

For a Life Force Theatre to take place, someone has to be a conduit or transmitter of the shaking. This is the role of the ecstatic shaman, the master of the universal life force, the interlocutor of spirited expression, the priest or priestess of the shaking, the captain of the spirit, or the energy director of a life force performance. Whether in the Kalahari, the mountains of China, the deep forests of the Amazon, the villages of the Caribbean, the sanctified Holy Ghost churches, or an experimental ecstatic theater, someone must step forth as a lightning rod and a conductor to bring down the lightning so it may be passed on to others.

One example of this kind of conducting takes place with one of the great qigong masters of our time, Grandmaster Jin-fa Zhang. One of his students and a colleague of mine, Rob Grace, writes about some of his learning experiences with the grandmaster:

> Every new student who comes to class gets the same treatment. Jin pulls you into his living room as you struggle to get your shoes off, all the while making loud kuhs and cracks and clucking like a disappointed mother. He then puts you in a standing posture, hits your spine a few times, and says "Good, good." When you finally compose yourself and look around, there's five or six other people in a variety of postures and hand mudras, moaning, crying, shaking, groaning, spinning in circles, and generally acting in ways one

might see in a nuthouse. To this day, the main form of communication between Jin and [me] is energy. I do not speak Shanghai-ese and he does not speak English. We barely make eye contact. From what I'm told, Jin was taught without talk as well. You were put in a position and left to your own devices. Proximity to the teacher alone was enough to spark your qi engine. Jin is much more accommodating. He enjoys seeing everyone lighten up and is quick to explode with qi. We call him the James Brown of qigong.

As we have seen in this book, the experiences reported by Rob Grace also take place in the Life Force Theatres of the Bushman shamans, in the Japanese practice of seiki jutsu, in the sanctified African American church, with the historical Shakers and Quakers, in kundalini practices, and in numerous other cultural ways throughout the world. It is a performed and experienced teaching that cannot be learned through words, but rather is transmitted only through shaking. We sometimes say it is an "energy teaching" or an "energy work," but "energy" is a hypothesized notion to account for the body performance of vibrations, trembling, quaking, and shaking, along with all the other ecstatic forms of movement. Yes, it feels like "energy" or "power" or "electricity," but it is the movement and shaking itself that unambiguously performs before an observer.

I will now present some testimonies of individuals who received the shaking medicine from me so you can have an even clearer idea of how it can be experienced. The first account is from Kenneth Cohen, teacher and healer of qigong and author of the classic text *The Way of Qigong: The Art and Science of Chinese Energy Healing,* among other works:

I had a personal experience of Brad's shaking power at the 1997 Common Boundary Conference on healing and spirituality in Washington, D.C. Brad Keeney and I had both been invited to present lectures. Although we had not been introduced, as soon as our eyes met, we recognized each other. We walked immediately toward each other and embraced with a simultaneous exclamation of "Brother!" My wife was standing nearby and was astonished to see me enthusiastically renew a friendship with a stranger! Brad and I had what the Chinese call *yuan fen,* "destined affinity."

On the last day of the conference, Brad asked me if he could give me a "gift from the Kalahari." Although I didn't know what he had in mind, I accepted. Brad and I found a quiet corner of the hotel. He placed one of his hands on my upper back and the other opposite on my upper chest. He began to shake vigorously and apparently involuntarily throughout his entire body. His face, shoulders, torso, and feet were vibrating with some invisible power, like a wave that was continuously cresting in his body and crashing and rippling in his fingertips. I felt the trembling power pass through me. Brad whispered African prayers in my ear, which I knew were prayers of blessing and protection.

While receiving this beautiful "gift," I was transported to the Kalahari. I saw the tribal people with whom he had danced; I viewed their villages and landscape. I was in Africa as truly as if I had opened my eyes and found myself physically there.[2]

Connie Forbister, who had been a friend of Cree holy man Grandfather Albert Lightning, was codirector of the Weechi-It-Te-Win Residential Youth Program in Fort Frances, Ontario, Canada. She tells her experience with the shaking medicine:

I went to see Brad in May, 1994, because I had hives and sore legs and wanted to be doctored. I went to his place with my husband, my boss, and his wife. I gave him an offering and we talked. I then told him why I had come and described a dream about a man I knew who had died a couple of years ago. As Brad began shaking, I knew he had no way of knowing anything about this man, but he interrupted me and asked whether this guy makes jewelry. Brad told me that he was visioning a silver necklace with a particular black stone and sure enough, there was such a necklace, just as Brad described it. In fact, the guy who I dreamed about, the man name Jim Brass who had died, was a jewelry maker. He did make a silver necklace with a black stone in it. He made it for his wife and I always wanted it. I knew she would give it to me if I now asked for it.

When Brad shakes with you, it overwhelms you when it first starts. You can feel it right away. It touches you deeply. What happens in a ceremony is that there is a lot of action going on. In such a situation I go into a trance-like state and I really don't remember a lot of what happens during the actual doctoring. I can remember Brad chanting, drumming, and rattling. After he doctored me, my sore legs and hives cleared up. I felt like I had been in a sweat lodge or a serious ceremony that lasted much longer than it actually did. I felt refreshed and healthy, mentally as well as physically. I haven't forgotten it. In fact I think about it a lot. When I get a chance, I will ask Brad for some more doctoring for other things.

There is a powerful thing happening with his medicine. I have never seen anything like it before. I've been around a lot of healers and medicine people and this one is pretty wild and powerful! He is interesting and decent. Anyone can go to him—it doesn't matter what color (or creed) you are.

Another member of the American Indian community, Charlie Monkman, a Cree, also talks about his experience:

I went to visit Brad. He is uncanny the way he is in tune with the spirits. I imagine that the gifts this man has would be seen as unreal by people who live solely with a scientific worldview. My role in my culture is very specific—I help the medicine people who do this work, helping them get the sacred things they need, like different parts of the plants and animals. When he shook with me, the room was totally dark, but I could see those little lights flying around all over the place. I've seen them before in sweat lodges. They are not lights that shine through some tiny holes through the darkness. I truly believe it is some sort of energy that is present. I could hear Brad talking in some kind of other language.

It was wild. I've been doctored before and know some powerful medicine people since I've been on this road, this search for the spirits. After we finished, Brad looked really different. I felt different. I felt heavy when we started and I felt very light when we were finished. He looked like he had finished running a marathon.

Before going to him I never ever dreamed. At most I might have one dream a year that I couldn't remember. After my experience with Brad, I have been dreaming every night and remembering all of my dreams. I had some phenomenal and fantastic dreams that same evening. It was like I was flying out of my body over the grounds . . . it was unbelievable and it was so clear I was almost frightened. I then had clear visions of my life as how I grew up as a little boy. I could remember everything about my life, whereas I couldn't before because of the pain I grew up with. It was just phenomenal. It's been that way ever since my time with him.

Here is a description from a social worker who experienced the shaking medicine:

The shaking and vibration were very gentle at first but as I surrendered, it became very intense and my thirst for union with spirit shifted from fear to an indescribable passion. . . . It was fluid beauty without description—velvet nothingness. . . . It both grounded me and elevated me simultaneously—like the sky being wrapped around the earth. As the energy vibrated through every cell and vein in my body, I felt two things at once—an unspeakable thirst to live in spirit and yet an equal passion to serve others and let the healing energy flow like a river into others . . . as I surrendered to the shaking, my fears melted away in human sweat and fire (the heat generated by Brad's body is hotter than the coals in a sweat lodge). . . . At one point I remember feeling a tidal wave of strength, pushing my arms forward and entering into the soul of the universe. I was rocked with the beauty and violence of the world.

A psychotherapist reports:

I felt a lot of pressure in my head. I felt that pressure for an hour or two after I left. I felt good though I was so dizzy with the whole experience, I couldn't remember anything to say so I let sounds and words just come out. I left feeling full and good. I was a little high and happy. I have been on other spiritual experiences, including my vision quest, but when I came home I felt disappointed and let down. I did not experience that this time. Instead I felt peace. I felt I had received something very important and precious to my life.

On September 25, 1994, Jesse Abbot, a teacher of English literature and composition, met me in a Manhattan apartment. He wrote about his shaking experience:

Laughter was the healing force that defined the beginning of this encounter. . . . I then decide to find out about this work. A mild energy is first born [in me] though I see that Keeney is already drenched with sweat, shaking a lot. I am in the chair now, and die in this chair. Limp. Weight of hand or chin in the dark on my limp head. There are more urgent vocalizations from Keeney now, alternately gentle and wrathful. Cleansing wailing. Goading, urgent, insistent. Calling to a child. Suggesting that I answer in kind. . . . There are loud, right-at-the-ears-immediate bells, bear-held on both sides. . . . I am able finally to wail, celebrating goodness everywhere and mourning my own and others' suffering. Something snaps in my spine, and with it, a "final" death. I fall even more limp in the chair, release all hostility and fear period, and trust completely in the very essence of whatever stalks me. The essence will not harm me. . . .

Now we are somehow on equal ground. I have a disciplined rush of compassion in my belly that spreads as energy outward, and I guide Keeney's hands, my eyes closed, in a carefully executed series of movements, sensing he is guiding me in much the same way. . . .

When things are over, I realize that a lot of light must have been spinning through this room. I had my eyes closed most of the time, but for hours afterward I have after-images of something shining in my eyes, whether they are opened or closed. . . . I am feeling that something related to light in general has been given back to me.

Finally, I offer a personal account written by Nor Hall, Ph.D., an archetypal psychologist, playwright, and the author of *The Moon and the Virgin, Those Women,* and *Broodmales:*

I am working in my office around the corner from Brad Keeney's house when an extraordinary clap of thunder and strike of lightning clearly signals the end of the therapy hour. It happens at 2:55. Later that afternoon I talk with Keeney about the problem of language—what words work to describe what he does, which reminds me to ask him what he had been doing at 2:55 in the afternoon. He asks if I am asking about the thunder. He was in his altar lighting his pipe. The fire crackled in the bowl, sparks leapt, and the black clouds crashed. I couldn't see anything in the vicinity that had been literally struck, but I am struck, once again, by the way he moves in tune with the natural world. Perhaps many of us do, but the difference is that when he is around, you are always on the lookout for it.

Unlike traditional shamans, Keeney belongs to no tradition. Every tradition he comes into contact with wants to claim him, but he's driving right off the world cliff into the sunset. Every time he steps into his altar room and closes the door he is the sun going down into its nighttime passage. The lights go out. Sound swells. There are three of us crammed into a space like a cupboard. A rattle lights up. A divebombing firefly. Its iridescence is made more uncanny by its radar like moves. We are so close together in the dark, but it speeds by without ever hitting us. Accoutrements of Keeney's vocation pack the space: carved antlers, painted drum, tobacco, the piece of sacred pipe. Not only Native implements of spirit work, there are African seeds, animal skins, a bird's nest, painted rocks, feathers, cloth, paintings, an image of Christ, the candle (now out). I can't see anything but the green light of the vibrating rattle. The air is charged. It is the electricus of silk rubbed amber. The same sort of charge that makes my hair stand on end a week later in a violent storm on the North Shore of Lake Superior. The rattle's shaking aerates the room. The sounds emanating from Keeney reverberate my eardrums. In an instant our configuration is changed. Our friend with the back pain is sitting. I had been pressed against his knee with my back to the curtained door, but I am suddenly swept on to Keeney's back and feel a bear's growl move deeply through me and out my finger tips which have been placed forcefully onto my friend's head. Keeney drums his fingers on my head and blows word-fragments into our ears. It is loud and wild, then alternately quiet and close. I don't know what a transmission is, but I can feel that something from elsewhere/elsewhen has powerfully rearranged us in relation to each other.

Although he has the tools of a shaman's trade (the drum, etc.), it appears he doesn't need anything but the instrument of his own body. His body is played: knocked and swayed, sung and spun. Put through the legendary hoops. The energy that moves him in extraordinary ways seems to be readily accessible in ordinary moments. The boundary between states is instantly soluble. I notice also that being in his presence has a way of dissolving the bundling boards that people erect to keep themselves separate. His work/art makes us a tribe. As to the training he hasn't had: systemic psychotherapy has a lot less to do with getting him here than having been a Baptist, ball player, and a jazz pianist. All modes of spiritual kinesthesia.

Because of an unselfconscious talent for the mercurial, he can shape shift in response to perceived need. He is a mobile shaman, (like therapists in New York who provide in-car service between home and office). Instead of staying in a particular hut and requiring that the people come walking in a particular way, purify themselves in a particular manner, and respond according to a shared cultural pattern, he has no idea what will transpire once the vibration gains momentum. Each encounter generates an original composition. To the rational personality his moves appear utterly wild and unpredictable because he is listening with an interior apparatus that picks up messages from dreams, the environment, weather, objects, birds, etc. It's not a guessing game with him. He's entirely focused, but on non-rational events.

His vitality rubs off in various ways. In my case it snapped the lid off a dusty Native Grandmother doll full of unconscious treasure. I started writing a novel, talking to strangers, making things with my hands, and receiving a voluminous and welcome rush of dreams. Call it by whatever name, like "shamanic contact-improv," contact with him shakes up a life.

I would like to modify Nor Hall's comment and say that it is contact with "shaking" that shakes up a life. It shook up mine, and it can shake up yours. And that is a good thing! All of the experiences that these people report are also found, as this book has demonstrated, in past and present cultures where shaking is honored and performed. There is nothing special about the shaker. It is the shake that is the tonic, medicine, and elixir.

The shake is like the wind. It blows through every spot on Earth. If you are ready for it, it can move you and take you somewhere. I invite you to be part of a new revolution, a coming-of-age of the human body with its fullest range of expression. Don't wait to learn what you need to know. Instead, be immediately available for the spirit to move you. Be on hand for life to shake you. The universe has always been ready for you. You are the one who needs to say, "I'm here to rock and roll!"

I always infuse each Life Force Theatre with heavy doses of light frivolity and a sense of the absurd. It serves as a kind of inoculation to protect us from being too serious about the unbelievable experiences that the shaking medicine can deliver. We certainly don't want to have the kind of a revolution, within ourselves or across the globe, that lasts only for a moment. Remember the historical lesson taught by the

Quakers who lost their quake and the Shakers who lost their shake. Let the spiritual gifts, whether visionary, energetic, or otherwise, come and go. See the letting go as a spiritual cleansing that empties you for the next round of shaking. If you don't let go, you'll get attached to the spiritual gifts and find that you want even more of them. This spiritual materialism leads to the kind of excess that eventually collapses from its own weight.

What the shake teaches is that all we can ever count on is change. Everything changes, including the way things change. The paradox is this: What we want to hold on to and cherish the most can be held only if we allow it and our relationship with it (along with ourselves) to never stop changing. When we are most fully alive, we are shape-shifters, changing all the ways we can be alive. Our bodies will shift and shake, as will our understandings and habits of action. The more we change, the more we become who we were meant to be. Or restated in our new understanding: The more we shake, the more we are alive. Become the wind, the ocean, the sky, and the land. Become inseparable from the ever-changing and ever-morphing Earth.

What follows is a task you should perform when you are ready to say yes to the shaking medicine:

Purchase the most interesting saltshaker you can find. Bring it home and create an altar for it, surrounding it with gifts and sacred things. Call this the "altar of shaking." It can be as small as a shoebox, and if you want, you can hide it underneath your bed. Now, thumb through this book and find five sentences that move you in a special way. Write down each sentence on a piece of paper, then cut the sentences into tiny pieces. When this has been done, place these pieces inside your saltshaker. Notice that they are too large to ever fall out.

Fantasize that a spirited essence will invisibly fall out of the shaker whenever you shake it. But this essence can be created only if you keep the shaker in your altar and honor it on a daily basis. Think about it and all the words it holds, doing so throughout the day. Sing to it at night, say a prayer for it, tell it a funny story or joke, tease it, and, most importantly, every once in a while, replenish it. Replenish by selecting five new sentences from this book, and again make tiny pieces that will replace the previous ones.

Now carefully consider this: You are a shaker. You are filled with all kinds of pieces of information, experiences, resources, talents, gifts, abilities, sufferings, meanings, strategies of action, dreams, and feelings. If you can find a way to place the whole of your life inside the altar of the great mystery, and if you honor the shaker that is you, then when you shake, a magical essence will be delivered. The gods are waiting for you to sanctify your life as a shaker, a vessel ready for mixing and delivering the sacred wisdom and blessings to all who are fortunate to know you.

STAGING A LIFE FORCE THEATRE

When you have committed yourself to becoming a shaker and want to host your own Life Force Theatre, you can begin by following a ritual protocol that helps you bring forth spirited experience. The Kalahari Bushmen typically dance once a week, sometimes more and sometimes less. You can choose to perform the Life Force Theatre whenever you feel the need for inspiration and revitalization, perhaps once a week, more or less, like the Bushmen. Keep in mind that any structure also carries with it a risk of losing improvisational inspiration—that is, a response-ability to the changes that are called forth in each unique situation and moment. I find the following stages to be useful considerations for structuring a Life Force Theatre, though I recommend maintaining a readiness to be open to any instantaneous change, so that spontaneity and improvisation are freely permitted to express themselves.

Stage One: Establishing an Enhanced Sacred Context
At the start of each performance of the Life Force Theatre, bring forth everything that can possibly enhance the ceremonial context in ways that activate and deepen faith, spiritual longing, compassion, worship, and a reaching out for the divine. Rather than reducing and simplifying a ceremony to a few vital ingredients (like monotonous drumming, body

postures, hyperventilation, or trance procedures), I suggest working in the opposite direction: making the setting as sacred and religious in tone as possible. Do so with an attitude of ecumenical acceptance while having readily available doses of play and merriment. The setting needs to evoke the sacred, but without any unnecessary limitation of creativity and appropriate playfulness.

Music and rhythmic preludes that evoke a sense of mystery help set up a sacred context. Incense, chanting, sacred images, and storytelling further contribute to opening the stage for shamanic experience and transformation. I sometimes have people set up a temporary altar for the occasion, adorning it with things they gather in the local ecology or from dream images that are personally important to the participants. One of the most vital contributions the facilitator(s) can make in this preparatory stage is to share her personal spiritual experiences, particularly those that led her to bring together the ceremonial gathering. In this regard, I typically mention the names of my spiritual teachers and share a few stories of my times with them, as well as talk about some of my own visions and experiences, and then ask others to share some of their own spiritual stories. This discourse effectively sets the mood for the shaking work.

Stage Two: Shaking the Words and Meanings

Once a sacred context is set up, it may carry the liability of bringing forth too much seriousness and reverence, which results in a diminished desire for creative play. Stage two is an invitation to assume the trickster attitude. Here I become a jester, teasing and laughing about the absurdity of life and the very occasion that has brought us together. Jokes and enactments of the absurd, along with inspired utterance of nonsense, mark the expression of this period. Contrary to some people's expectation, this phase actually helps deepen the sacred context, while helping free it from the kind of unnecessary piety that can disrupt a full flight into ecstatic shaking.

The words, meanings, and logically framed expectations that people bring to the ceremony are shaken in this stage of the Theater. I sometimes ask every person to provide one word that expresses his or her most important hope for the ceremony. For example, one group set forth the following list:

Shaking	Rebirth
Love	Vision
Ecstasy	Know
Healing	Surrender
Connection	Joyful
Peace	Play
Dance	Transformation
God	Creation
Creativity	Truth

I then ask someone to shout out a word, brought forth without deliberate thought, a word that comes straight from the unconscious mind with no necessary logical connection to what we are doing. In the particular situation I just described, someone shouted out "Rhinoceros." The list is then used to generate a free-associative talk, weaving the list of words together to spin a kind of speech that flows without conscious purpose or rational direction. For instance, in this case I said:

"We have gathered here today to bring forth the *shaking love* that delivers *ecstasy* and *healing* to all those who make the Big *Connection*. I am talking about reaching out for the gentle arms of *peace* that bring us into a *dance* with *God*. Here we will awaken a *creativity* that enables a *rebirth* of the *vision* that we were born to *know* and carry with us throughout every day of our life. To make these things happen, we must fully *surrender* to the *joyful play* that transforms all of life, a *transformation* that was initiated at the beginning of *creation*. In its *truth* we find that we are related and inseparable from all things, with the sky, the great waters, and the land. We learn that we are even a brother and sister to the *rhinoceros,* whose horn aims and proclaims our entry into the sacred heavens."

With this performance of creative improvisation, a fresh sense of "aliveness" is brought into the room that promises the forthcoming of creative ceremonial transformation. There are many ways to play and improvise at this stage. What is important is that people feel that the situation is "coming alive."

Stage Three: Invocation

Here, the leader or facilitator first makes a simple announcement as to how everyone should enter into the shaking ceremony. The goal is to try to help free everyone from preconceived notions and attachments to overly specified outcomes. I usually say something like this:

"There is no right way to shake. It doesn't matter whether you shake gently or strongly, with rhythm or without rhythm. It is more important for you to be as free as possible of any attachment to form or any expectation of outcome. Release your desire to set forth any idea of what you want to take place. We are not here to dance. Dance implies a recognized form, something that is beautiful and readily identifiable as a work of choreography. We are here to go past dance. Dance a little, if you are so called, but then release the dance. Fall into the movements that are past the territory of dance.

"Hand yourself over to your deepest unconscious mind, to the unseen gods and to their transformative winds of change. Tinker, experiment, and play with your mind and body, doing so to help open yourself to a new possibility. This is your laboratory, your playground, your sandbox, your temple, your church, your altar, your ceremony, your theater, a place for the whole of your body-mind-soul.

"Consider trying anything and be ready for all movement. Move in order to trip yourself out of any habits you have brought with you. Make yourself ready to be grabbed by the spirit. Be comfortable with all unexpected outcomes whether they are a deeper stillness or an erratic jump. It doesn't matter whether you are still or whether you shout. There is no right way to be in this moment. There is only making yourself available to the medicine that is present in the air you breathe. The spirit is here and continues to arrive as we show ourselves to be ready for it."

I then proceed to make an invocation or prayer, usually beginning with words and moving to the improvisation of heartfelt sounds. I typically am drumming as I voice this calling forth of the spirits. My drumming is not repetitive in an unaltered way, but instead is rhythmically changing, often syncopated, and flowing in relationship to what is said and sounded.

Stage Four: Rhythms (and/or Music) for Shaking

Now it is time to initiate the rhythms and/or music for shaking. You may wish to use the CD that accompanies this book. At times I mix its rhythms with other recordings of sacred music, doing so with a live DJ. I also use live musicians and percussionists to accompany the recorded rhythms or allow the performance to be completely improvisational. As a drummer and keyboardist, I am typically part of the rhythmic production. What matters is that the rhythms are wild and not monotonous. Shaking medicine is more activated by ever-changing rhythms that evoke ecstasy rather than by the monotonous rhythms that are more suitable for light trance induction.

This stage usually lasts an hour or less, depending upon when it feels "done." During the shaking period, the facilitator can bring different people together, facilitate movement by gentle touch, make rhythmic sounds, chant incantations, and improvise in any way that is appropriate and relevant.

Stage Five: Mystical Incubation

When the rhythms stop, everyone is asked to lie down or sit and close their eyes. Soft and inspiring music may be played in the background. The facilitator announces an invitation to enter into mystical incubation, saying something like:

"The shaking has cleaned your heart and made you ready for a mystical lesson. You have been emptied and are prepared for communion and communication with spirit. Perhaps the lesson will be one of continued vibrations. Or maybe it will be taught through a feeling or a word or sound or even something you see with your mind's eye. As you lie down, know that you are available for being led by spirit. Make a simple request or prayer for help. It may be specific or general or as simple as 'Guide me and teach me' or 'May Thy will be done.' It is unimportant whether your conscious mind is aware of the teaching that will now take place. It may be given quietly and invisibly and delivered to your unconscious mind and show up later in the day or week as a surprising thought, feeling, action, or special dream. Do not be concerned as to how the spirit will teach you. Simply allow spirit to teach you in its own way."

During this time of mystical incubation, the facilitator may walk around the group, making improvised and whispered sounds if that seems fitting. One may also make clapping sounds from time to time, or simply remain silent. The facilitator must remain available for the spirit to move in whatever ways seem natural and appropriate for this stage.

Stage Six: Community Sharing

At this stage, invite people to get up, stretch, and, for those who wish to do so, become ready to share their experiences and stories. This sharing provides an opportunity for further shaking work—as experiences are shared, rhythms and sounds may be reintroduced and people may find themselves having additional shaking of their bodies. Or everyone may remain still without further ecstatic performance. This time should allow for anyone to make a contribution and, at the same time, allow for further improvisation of the spirit. When the sharing is completed, it is good to reintroduce humor and play some joyous music as people move about. This is also an appropriate time to have food and beverages as a celebration of what took place.

Keep in mind that these stages are suggestions and do not have to be rigidly followed. Any part may be changed or sequenced in a different order. For example, before the shaking commences, the facilitator may ask the participants to silently or publicly voice what each person wants to focus on, whether it is a specific or general request for transformation or spiritual blessing. I personally prefer that people be less conscious of their desires before shaking, allowing themselves to be as empty as possible. What you think is important in your life may change (or be made more obvious) after shaking.

The key to making the shaking medicine strong and meaningful is to encourage improvisation and allow it to move with the flow of spirit. Shaking medicine surrounds itself with joy and love; it is not sanctimonious and overly serious, though the most powerful moments of shaking may be the most profound experiences of one's life. The Life Force Theatre is an improvisational theater of the wild, a place for spirit to soar into unexplored heights of ecstasy.

Over the years I have moved away from seeing this work primarily as a context for physical and mental (and spiritual) healing, although those outcomes may take place. I prefer seeing it as a theater that aims to inspire people's lives. Joyful shaking is as powerful as one's heart is able to open to love. As you open to the flow of divine love, the psyche and soul are cleansed and made available for spiritual gifts and lessons. These, in turn, inspire one to bring forth creative expression, whether through music, words, imagery, or other forms of performance and creation. In a way, the Life Force Theatre is an incubator for hatching one's creativity, for inspiring one's desire to be a vibrant part of life, and for feeling renewed and connected to the whole of life. Of course, these outcomes contribute to healing, recovery, health, and well-being.

Stage Seven: Shaking the Mind with Shamanic Conversation

In this final stage of the Life Force Theatre, I announce that the ecstatic shaking of bodies experienced in the first part of the theater was a cleansing, an emptying, a readying for another kind of shaking medicine—a shaking the mind so as to loosen and release one's inner gifts, talents, and creative expression. I ask for volunteers who have felt inspired by their experience with soulful body shaking in the Life Force Theatre and want to do something with it.

I invite them to have an unusual kind of conversation with me, what I call a *shamanic conversation,* whose purpose is to shake their mind and help unleash their creative presence in life. A shamanic conversation is a transformational encounter that helps them utilize their inspiration toward producing some form of creative expression. I may encourage participants to paint an image, orchestrate a dance, write a story, perform an unusual ritual, wear a hidden message, enact a social intervention, or incubate a dream in an unexpected fashion, to mention just some of the possibilities. Here the process uses the inspiration brought forth by body shaking as a compass pointing toward a unique journey into personal creativity. The Life Force Theatre not only helps people to be inspired, but also facilitates finding their unique way of creatively participating in the world.

I believe that all forms of effective healing and transformation that are mediated through conversation and social interaction are existentially absurd and are often misled and short-circuited by assumptions regarding the importance and/or priority of rationality and conscious awareness in the construction of experiential reality. The dilemmas and paradoxes of human beings derive from the multifaceted and constantly shifting nature of experience. The idea that we enact linear historical narratives organized by logical premises contradicts the irrational and illogical ways we interact with others, make decisions, and construe meanings. The limitations of conscious mind and abstraction simply provide impoverished material for transformational work. In particular, psychological understanding, while capable of entertaining the contemplative mind, is typically unable to radically change anyone's habits of action and interaction.

Shamanic conversation is an alternative to the addictive search for psychological understanding and privileged meanings. Shamanic conversation is the spoken and enacted performance of "trickster shamanism" and is historically supported by therapists who espoused experientially oriented practices of absurd psychotherapy. Shamanic conversation proposes that more unconscious process and creative imagination be brought into human encounter. Here the unconscious is regarded as a vital source of irrational wisdom and a necessary presence and co-guide in the transformational process.

The complexity of neuronal interaction and social interaction makes a comprehensive understanding of human behavior and experience technically impossible. The consequence of fully apprehending this cognitive limitation is a revolutionary understanding: namely, that theories of psychology (and simplistic renderings of spirituality, including naive shamanism) are absurd fictions that are largely irrelevant to the inspired performance of everyday life. Faced with the unknowable and unrealizable complexity of experience, we are wise to loosen our attachment to overarching psychotherapies and psychologies that assume to understand the existential situation and then proceed to prescribe stereotyped action.

Instead, we can follow the orientation of the improvising cultural tricksters. Rather than "knowing" before "acting," they suggest that "we act in order to know." Continuing with this form of interactive presence, the more surprising and unexpected the act, the more likely previously unseen things will be revealed. This "jumping headfirst into the water" approach suggests that a shamanic conversational encounter embraces a more open improvisational stance, always ready to change course and proceed on the basis of the circumstances and experiential outcomes at hand. The wild conversations of trickster shamanism are presented as an alternative to the overly rational practices of psychotherapy and the overly psychological ways of routinized spiritual and shamanic healing.

The basic ideas underlying shamanic conversation include an emphasis upon calling forth unconscious (typically irrational) sources of communication and expression and allowing them to steer the course of transformational interaction. Dreams and the creative arts are fully utilized in this orientation, as are specific ways of introducing nonsense and enactments of the absurd. Shamanic conversation fully brings back the important role of the cultural trickster. Its purpose is to help people trip themselves out of their overly conscious minds and habits and fall into unexpected, though desired, changes, rather than leading them into trivial, often non-effectual fantasies of insight or reasoned prescriptions of action designed to eradicate troublesome behaviors and interactions.

Part of the shamanic conversational art of effective transformation and growth is juggling and shaking frames of meaning, whether introducing unexpected contextual frames or pulling out the rug from beneath any received view of things. The conversational methods of wildly shifting contexts are a sleight-of-hand-and-mouth work that juggles the frames that give meaning to lives. The goal is to move from impoverished frames (the presenting communications about suffering) to resourceful frames that accentuate the natural gifts, abilities, and magical resources of people and their situation.

Nowhere is the creativity of change making, whether with individuals or with groups, more evident than in unexpected prescriptions for future action. Any effort to help another person change without radical recommendations for alternative performances of change is potentially impotent and unethical. Trickster ethics and shamanic responsibility require a full allegiance to the callings of the deep wild and to the paradoxical wisdom held in the directive: "To know yourself, change!"

The essence of existential transformation involves working the underlying existential dichotomies, distinctions, and dualities that hold a person's suffering and symptomatic experience. The juggling of these dichotomies so as to transcend their "either/or" locked-in structure may be regarded as a shamanic dialectic. The Zen use of *koans* and experiential dilemmas suggests that irrational and unconsciously inspired wild interaction with a person's dilemma not only provides an escape from its tormenting grip, but also utilizes the problem at hand to empower a new direction of personal growth. This process constitutes the truest meaning of "spiritual prosperity": transforming existential suffering into the alchemical gold of joy and bliss.

Shaking medicine may be seen as using automatic, reflexlike responses of the body to orchestrate a psychodrama of shamanic transformation. With one part of the body enacting inner unconscious wisdom, other parts enact the present dilemmas and existential dichotomies. In the shaking there is a spontaneous choreography that precipitates kinesthetic trance and mind-in-body resolutions. Here we find that a person's authentic self is nothing less than his or her body.

The problems, symptoms, and sufferings of human beings can be recast as the unconscious callings for personal and social transformation. Seen this way, the problem is a lighthouse pointing to the direction of change. Implicitly acknowledging its importance and uncommon wisdom, the change agent of shamanic conversation enters the wilderness of the unconscious. There reside unexpected shifts of meaning, fantasies, metaphors, and irrational enactments of the absurd. Like shamans of old who enter the wilderness to find healing for their constituents, the wild conversationalist (and talking shaman) enters the unconscious wilderness of the social situation, lying in wait for the curing and healing that unfolds naturally and without reason, unavailable to the understanding of anyone. It is the unconscious and its invitation to enter into the wildness of our imagination that brings forth change and growth.

The past and present proliferation of professionalized orientations to healing, body therapies, shamanisms, and psychotherapies always bring forth prohibitions and orthodoxies that threaten the presence of creative sensitivities and imagination. I call for multiple renderings of conversational anarchy, suggesting that authentic change and growth of the psyche, soul, relationship, and sociocultural ecology are not possible without the winds of creative freedom.

With a challenge to all orthodoxies, I ask for renewed interest and curiosity in how ignorance and humility, rather than expertise and professionalism (and political correctness), can revitalize the practice of everyday transformational work. We need shamanic directives aimed at shaking, freeing, and inspiring the imagination of today's people helpers. Everyone needs to be reminded that we are all in the same position as those who seek help—lost in the cosmos, hoping for meanings we can never find and plotting liberating action that seems just outside the reach of reason. The only way out is through the irrational and unconscious wilderness.

Shaking medicine, whether administered by shaking bodies or shaking conversations, abandons the ideas, understandings, and practices of psychotherapy and spirituality. It goes beyond the role of a therapist or spiritual teacher. Instead, one becomes more like a voice coach or a teacher of theater, painting, or sport. The aim is to awaken a person's inspiration and inner gifts as a performer on the stage of life. Finding your unique gift and becoming inspired to bring it forth is the most transformative experience. This alone can tune all the other aspects of our life, from how we relate to others to how we choose to manage the activities of each day.

What people are looking for is not problem-solving (life is not a problem that can be solved) or spiritual growth (your soul is already fully grown and waiting for you to notice it). Everyone wants to be inspired and to find the unique talent he or she has to express his or her inspiration. The Life Force Theatre and all the traditions of shaking ecstasy are primarily about this awakening of each person's creativity.

When we find our unique voice and are inspired to express it, we meet each moment of the day in a fully prepared way. In this manner, our hearts are full of passion and our souls are awakened to respond. Our mind becomes obedient, a servant, to the higher calls of creativity rather than being a cranky authority that tries to bully us through each personal moment and social interaction with self-righteous (and overly assertive) posturing.

The Life Force Theatre aims to awaken hearts and serve the mission of our soul. It harnesses mind to be under the influence of love rather than power. This work is fully aligned with all the expressive arts and sees them as inseparable from spirited religion and the performance of everyday life. The Life Force Theatre is more than a once-a-week performance. It has the potential to expand and embrace each day. As experienced shakers learn, the shaking medicine can go with you, ready to be drawn upon whenever needed, whether as an inner vibration unseen by others or as a vibrant expression spontaneously exhibited (and perfectly situated) in a social milieu. Welcome to the stage of the Life Force Theatre. Over time, it will become the grand stage for the performance of the rest of your life.

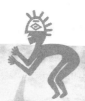

11

THE ULTIMATE MEDICINE

From Shaken Faith to Shaking Faith

My shaking began over thirty-six years ago and arrived in the form of an overwhelming mystical experience. Since that time, I have spent practically every day of my life wondering about the mysteries of shaking and the transformational consequences associated with it. Through the Life Force Theatre, I observed people having every imaginable kind of ecstatic experience and expression. They rolled on the floors, went wild and crazy, had religious experiences, felt themselves being morphed into other physical shapes and realities, dropped to the floor in a deep state of trance, and had waking dreams, hallucinations, visions, deep calm and peace, creative discovery, artistic inspiration, healing from mental and physical illness, revitalization, and heightened abilities. If you can imagine it, it probably happened in the Life Force Theatre.

For me personally, I found the theater to be a wonderful experimental venue for learning about the many ways that vibrations and shaking can affect people. But all along the way, I felt that the cultural traditions that brought forth the shaking through devotion to and love of a Supreme Being facilitated the deepest and most satisfying ecstatic experiences. There, the spirit was more likely to be *in* most of the parishioners, whereas in the nonreligious theater, the spirit was more likely to be *on* most of the audience.

Over the years, I found myself less and less interested in a spirited theatrical performance and more and more longing to be in religious community with those within whom the spirit resides. With them, I celebrated the joy of being in the spirit. For years, I all but stopped performing the Life Force Theatre and emphasized more involvement in sacred settings. Not surprisingly, I found the shaking to be ecstatically powerful and beautifully transforming in all the world's religions I was fortunate enough to experience. But I found a special delight when I returned to the religious tradition I had grown up in. This did not mean that I held my religion of origin to be more true or better than the other religions. That view, I think, is an arrogance that is not justifiable. None of us has enough wisdom to make such a claim, though we can humbly say that we are inseparable from both our family of origin and our religion of origin (our most important beliefs, values, and practices). For some, their religion of origin is agnosticism, science, or a materialistic school of common sense. I don't see those worldviews as religions any less than my own. They don't inspire me, but who am I to judge whether they are a good fit for someone else? And if that was the person's religion of origin, then it is an inseparable part of who he or she is.

I will always be appreciative to Sam Gurnoe, the first medicine man who sat me on a cliff as part of a vision fast. He told me in a sweat lodge, "I pray that my cultural ways will help you empower and embrace your own cultural way." He didn't evangelize or push the superiority of his spirituality, but framed it as a relative of other traditions. By meeting one of your spiritual relatives, you may be encouraged to find your parents, knowing that the whole multigenerational family comes from one source.

My participation in many shaking traditions, inside and outside of religions, did in fact bring me home to the country-church services I grew up in. Let me immediately pause to say that I understand the resistance and allergies people have to religion. Seeing and hearing all the ways in which the loving presences of Jesus, Buddha, and Muhammad, among others, have been distorted is enough to make anyone sick and ashamed. Yet no matter how perverted a religion becomes, the originating inspirations remain as transformative today as they were in their beginning.

I learned from my African elders the importance of honoring and maintaining a living relationship to all of my ancestors. And because my ancestors practiced a certain faith, I honor them and spiritually reach them more intimately when I honor their faith. That is part of the reason I love to hear the old gospel songs and the old-time preaching (as long as they preach New Testament love freely available to everyone, rather than self-righteous condemnation of outsiders). These experiences remind me of being a child and of the strong feelings of affection I had within my family while growing up. I am lucky to have been blessed by wonderful grandparents and parents, all of whom led deeply religious lives. Anything that keeps alive the fire of that love is good for my life. This contributes to why I love the religion they taught me.

The adoration of religion hasn't always been the case for me. As a young adult, I cringed whenever I turned on the television and heard the consumer-distorted sermons of the entrepreneur evangelists. They had no connection to the messages of love, humility, forgiveness, and charity given every Sunday morning in my grandfather's and father's churches. Similarly, when I heard any politician use God's name to justify a war or nationalistic pride, it made me sick and angry. That anger extended to the religious words they used, and sometimes to the religion they embraced. I subsequently had nothing to do with any religion that was being used for propaganda and wrongdoing.

However, the praying in sweat lodges, the dancing in the Kalahari, the singing in the Amazon, and the contemplations of emptiness in Japan, among other experiences, opened me up and swept away my anger and disgust. They allowed the truths of all religions, particularly the one I grew up with, to surge through my whole being without resistance or distraction. I then was able to learn how religious faith is the ultimate medicine on Earth. Only the loving truths of the great religions are capable of bringing forth the most transformative trembling, quaking, and shaking.

Religion should not be seen as distinct from spirituality. Religion is the highest way of honoring the spirit. When you are truly spiritual (that is, the spirit is *in* you), you will love religions. This may be the best test of your spirituality. If you are repulsed by any tradition of faith, then you are deceiving yourself and others by saying that you are spiritual. When the spirit is in you, it thirsts for contact with religion. The scriptures and holy books become like an elixir, spiritual food or water that quenches your deepest thirst and hunger. It makes you happy to hear sacred literature. When you are deep inside the spirit, you feel compassion for those spiritual impostors who used to anger you. Yes, their deeds and actions and defamation of the holy way are disturbing, but they don't interfere with your love for the religion they are denigrating.

The greatest medicine on Earth is shaking faith. It arises out of a heart that loves all the religions of the world, including those that are agnostic, skeptical, and cynical. It sees any important system of belief as holding a piece of the truth. Each tradition has caught an aspect of the whole truth. When the shaking medicine gets inside you, an inner fire is lit that enables the light to shine on the partial truths of all revelations. As the wisdom becomes revealed, you walk each day with a burning fire that shines the luminous truths through your entire being. This makes you want to sing and shout with joy! And you do so, even within yourself when it is not socially appropriate to do so publicly. You become alive with spirit.

Shaking medicine will not make you a spiritual drug addict, but it will from time to time make you feel as high as you have ever felt. People more often than not leave their seiki benches and the Life Force Theatre with dilated pupils and a feeling of being intoxicated with the spirit. But this ecstatic experience affects everyday life in a very positive way. It motivates you to be fully involved with your conventional activities in the world, whether they comprise parenting, physical labor, office work, sports, social activism, or civic responsibilities. When the spirit is inside you, you become a revolutionary who fights for the freedoms of all living beings, particularly the right of life for Mother Earth. The spirit is a citizen of Gaia.

Phyllis Mack, professor of history at Rutgers University and author of *Visionary Women: Ecstatic Prophecy in Seventeenth Century Eng-*

land, studied historical accounts of ecstatic women of the early Quakers. She was struck to find how their ecstatic lives empowered their everyday social lives. They participated in charity work, petitioned Parliament, advocated for prison reform, and gave money to the poor.

One of these ecstatic and prophetic Quakers, Margaret Fell, declared:

> We are a people that follow after those things that make for peace, love and unity . . . and do deny and bear our testimony against all strife, and wars, and contentions . . . and our weapons are not carnal, but spiritual. . . . And so we desire, and also expect to have the liberty of our consciences and just rights and outward liberties, as other people of the nation. . . . Treason, treachery, and false dealing do we utterly deny; false dealing, surmising, or plotting against any creature upon the face of Earth, and speak the truth in plainness, and singleness of heart.[1]

When the spirit resides within, we take our stand for peace and justice for all. We do not usurp the holy books and twist their meanings to psychotically justify war and harm against others. We take a nonviolent stand with the strength of the inner spirit, as did Gandhi and Dr. Martin Luther King Jr., against the double standards and diabolical distortions of spiritual truth. We stand for the life force rather than the death force, and we advocate spiritual rather than carnal power.

The call is for the mystical husband and the mystical wife, the mystical neighbor and the mystical citizen. Only when the spirit resides within will we have the strength to stand against the greedy and nationalistic leaders and their empty-headed and empty-hearted followers. No one can be an ecstatic patriot and shaking warrior for planet Earth unless the spirit of Earth resides within him or her. The call of the wild is not only a call for the spirit; it is a call for newborn activism, a call that sees through the double-talk of propaganda, whether it be dressed as religious, political, or religio-politico-consumerist rhetoric.

The loss of the shake is a measure of how overly committed we have become to seeking the fantasy of being fully in control. When the shake reenters a culture, people become less controllable. The hierarchies of religion, education, art, and community are challenged when people start dancing themselves into deep states of experiential freedom. When the quaking bodies give rise to visionary experience, the authority of written generalizations is weakened. The most dangerous revolutions do not take place with nationalistic propoganda, economic threat, and gunfire. When all is said and done, what happens in non-peaceful overthrows is simply that the names change. The more politics changes, the more the hierarchical game remains unaltered. The rich remain rich and the poor remain poor, and the laws get even stricter about keeping everyone's bodies and personal expression in control.

The way to change the world, the most important revolution that will change hearts and souls, takes place when people start dancing in the streets and call for the lifting of our spirit. If you want to change things, start humming, singing, and whistling. Music in the air will bring down the seriousness that maintains the tyrant's climate of totalitarianism. Laugh to melt away the edge of fear. Sing and the moral enforcers are silenced. The greatest fear of despots and dictators is joy. Bring in the clowns, merry tricksters, and sacred fools, and watch the politicians get laughed out of office.

The spirited shaker lives to shake, exchange spiritual gifts, create, and laugh. Each is inseparable from the other. The visions inspire and direct us to live better lives with one another, while the shaking invigorates our whole being and makes us ready to live the everyday with creative passion. The shaking and quaking arise not only from the awe of beholding the sacred, but from the belly laughs that bring everything and everyone down to size. We laugh with each other and at ourselves. The absurdity of the human condition is celebrated with convulsing laughter. We shake when we laugh and laugh at the shaking. What could be more ridiculous than finding out that the greatest gift on Earth is to be found in shaking?

We have seen a wide range of historical documentation of the ways in which a shaking faith can transform a life and fill it with innumerable gifts. This way of living is not confined to one part of the world.

Cultures from all locations have found their way to the shaking. Unfortunately, it has become all but extinct for the technologically enriched peoples. But there is no reason for things to stay that way.

I have personally experienced practically every form of spirited expression and shaking described in this book, whether it was noted in an account of a historical Shaker or that of a Kalahari shaman. That has been my destiny—to live and know and teach these things. More importantly, I have met other people throughout the world who have also had these experiences. We have a fire in our hearts, and we walk with great devotion and passion for all the great religions of the world. We know that these grand traditions of faith are a medicine chest holding the most powerful elixirs and medicines. The oldest cultures of the world teach us that *medicine* is a word that is not limited to what you buy at a drugstore. To the ecstatic and spirited shamans, mystics, and medicine people, *medicine* is "spirit"—that which can transform our whole being. Prayer is a medicine, as is song and dance. In the universal clinic for the care of all souls, shaking faith, reborn and resurrected in love, is the greatest medicine of them all.

I have returned to the Life Force Theatre, but now I see it as a spirited church, a synagogue, temple, medicine lodge, dance circle, and sacred gathering. I also see it as a stage, social gathering place, concert hall, dance studio, human relations laboratory, experimental theater, interactional classroom, ecstatic club, blues room, shamanic playground, and spirited party. These days, I usually cannot help but bring that old-time blues-brothers religion into the shaking celebration of praise and joy. At the same time, I know that if I take any of this too seriously, the spirit may lose interest. We must dance in the tension between the nightclub and the chapel, the sacred and the profane, the light and the dark, God and the Devil, the aroused and the relaxed. In the midst of the contraries, we find momentary and eternal truths.

We now arrive at the secret of shaking. It is quite simple and straightforward: Whenever you pull two opposites apart but don't break the invisible relational string that connects them, the whole thing will start to vibrate and shake. Imagine pulling apart a tight spring or a row of coiled springs with handles on each end, like the exercise device found in gyms. Stretch it farther and farther. It will eventually reach a point where it takes all of your might to pull and hold it. As you pull it as far as you can and try to hold it with your outstretched arms, you will feel your muscles and the pulled springs start to tremble and shake. This pulling of opposites creates the necessary tension for the emergence of quaking and shaking.

Each of us embraces many distinctions, dualities, and opposites that comprise the possibilities of our experiential universe. These competing thoughts, feelings, and worldviews are held in our bodies. Sometimes we feel attraction for someone, and then we feel the opposite. There are times when we are angry with the ones we love the most. Or we feel let down when we get what we want, or feel both worried and excited when catastrophe is about to take place. These are only a few examples of the many paradoxes underlying the experiences of our lives.

In the theater of the everyday, we are kinesthetically pulled in all kinds of directions, especially when these polarities act out. Love versus hate, victory versus loss, health versus illness, life versus death, and joy versus suffering are a few of the dancing opposites. These are the stretched springs that lie coiled at the base of our lives. They are filled with energy that is ready to spring forth and shake us up.

There is no kundalini serpent lying at the base of our spine. No X-ray will reveal a snake residing inside our body. To make this assumption is to make an error of misplaced concreteness—mistaking an abstraction or metaphor for a concrete object. The bigger truth is that we sit upon a plenitude of coiled tensions, embodying the stretched distinctions that organize the tragedies and comedies of our lives. In these tensions, these sacred contraries, lies the universal life force. This is where the shaking resides and where it can be awakened; this is where shaking begins and where it returns. At the base are the distinctions that confront one another in a great cosmic struggle. This is the home of kundalini, n|om, qi, Holy Spirit, and the universal life force.

In the struggle between life and death, and all of its derivative dualities, is the shaking power (or shakti). If either side of a distinction is victorious and conquers the other side, then the shaking power is gone. We are only winning—that is, able to activate the shaking medicine—when we allow the contraries to go at it. We must be ready to die in order to be ready to live, free to hate in order to be able to love more deeply, free to lose ourselves in order to find who we are. The world of William Blake, with its contrary-driven creative force, is the same world as the kundalini serpent power of Bhujangini. Through the archetypal interaction of the masculine and the feminine, the eternal battle of the sexes, we find the bliss that is married to suffering.

The mighty war fought between all imagined opposites serves the greater peace. We are biologically and existentially alive due to the combating (and cooperating) tensions that give pulse to life. When we shake, we are extending, pushing, and pulling all of the components of our experiential universe, with all of their contraries, in a transforming way. When the tension is released, we dance one step of the medicine dance and bring forth the shaking that momentarily transcends and subsequently realigns the juxtapositions, making us a retuned (perpetually reborn) whole being. Then the tensions recoil themselves, making ready for the next step and shake. In the shaking of the contraries, we become Shiva and hold the hands of God. Transformed in this way, we are ready to move the world, and even more readied for the movements of the world.

I want you to sit at your bench the next time you practice seiki jutsu and imagine all the important dichotomies in your life. They may be health versus sickness, companionship versus loneliness, meaning versus an absence of meaning, feeling rested versus feeling tired, success versus failure, being light versus being heavy, or anything else that comes to you as significant. Now make these dichotomies as specific as possible. Spell them out so they define the particularities of your present situation. Right this very moment, ask yourself whether the most important dichotomy in your life concerns reaching and maintaining a desired weight versus being overweight, or wanting to find a significant companion to live with versus living alone, or getting your heart to feel alive and full of love again versus feeling cold and without passion. Or is there something else that organizes the dilemmas of your life?

Now bring your personal dilemma, with its two opposing sides, into awareness. Proceed to choose a spot on your body that you can imagine holding one side of the dilemma and another part of your body that holds the other side. For the sake of simplicity, start by having one hand pretend that it is holding one side—say, being overweight—while the other hand holds the correct weight. In this situation, you might even take a pen and actually write "overweight" on one palm and the desired weight on the other palm.

Imagine marking all of the dichotomies of your life on your body. As you move forward to start the automatic movements and bring on the shaking, imagine that all of these warring opposites are interacting and exploring various ways to work things out. As you move your body, mentally visualize, hear, or feel the opposite sides as they push and pull you. Know that progress will be made in this tension between the contraries of your life. The dynamic interactions help set into motion the very changes you need.

Here's a modified, perhaps better way to do the exercise: Choose the hand you think is better suited to hold the solutions and the wisdom you believe can help evolve your whole being. Now consider using the other hand as the depository of all the issues, dilemmas, problems, and struggles that make up your life. Proceed to move and shake, allowing the wisdom and the struggles to interact in this body enactment of your existential situation. You can even clasp your hands together and watch how this can stimulate wild movements. You can clap your hands and have them interact with each other in a wide array of possibilities. Hold them above you or on the ground, place them against a stone, splash water with them, direct music, or have them beat your chest. Let the two hands that hold your wisdom and suffering find many ways to interact and dance together.

Whenever you shake, whether sitting, lying down, or standing, consider it a pushing and pulling of the dichotomies of your life. Some of these dichotomies are general while others are specific. Some are true dilemmas, such as "Do I accept the offer or decline it?" "Should I move in with him or wait for someone else? "Should we retire or keep working?" "Should we do it now or later?" Imagine everything in your life that can be split into a choice, a dilemma, or a duality, and imagine it is in your body. Believe me, it is: Your body carries and embodies all the differences that organize your thinking and feeling. You are (that is, your body is) what you think and what you feel. You are the distinctions that push and pull you through each day and each night.

Now you can more fully appreciate both that shaking is caused by the tension between our inner opposites and that shaking helps bring forth a resolution to these tensions, conflicts, and dilemmas. Following a good shake, you will feel clearer about things; have more access to your inner resources, creativity, and intuition; and be better tuned to live a more healthy and successful life.

However, when you reenter the everyday, things will get coiled and stretched out again. You will wake up in the middle of the night, worrying about whether to do this or to do that. You will find the tension back again, ready to be shaken for another resolution and reattunement. This is how we are organized to live our lives. We need to vibrate and shake on a regular basis to keep the contraries moving toward progression—that is, to draw upon the energy of our crises so that it serves as the motor for our personal and relational growth.

This provides a unique way of understanding how suffering helps bring forth joy. As the structure of the African American church reveals, we must bring in the suffering, hand it over to the Lord, then dance, shake, and shout for joy. On a daily basis, we can sit down with our heavy load, setting forth all the tensions caused by the conflict between opposing sides, and allow them to be moved, shaken, and transformed into an ecstatic moment of personal growth. Our therapist, coach, and spiritual teacher are the transformative vibrations and shakes. Bring all that life has done to get you out of balance, and let the shaking rebalance you.

All experienced ecstatic shamans know that their shamanism is a "death and resurrection show." They allow their burdens, shortcomings, failures, illnesses, mistakes, sins, and crimes to bury them in the ground.

Shamans aren't afraid to see that they are no better than any criminal behind bars, and that no one is any better than or superior to any other living creature, whether it is a rat, snake, or insect. Understanding where we really are in the grand scheme of things humbles us in a good way, and helps us give up any arrogant notion that we are capable of winning any battle, internal or external, on our own. In this coming to terms with our true situation, we are leveled. Consequently, our self-importance experiences a momentary death. Overcome by the data, it surrenders and says, "I am nothing." In this existential death, the shaman sincerely reaches out to a greater wisdom, a higher being, and begs for help. "I surrender my soul to thee. Take me, make me, and shake me." These are prayers of surrender and requests for transformation.

This is when the biggest magic takes place. When we humble ourselves and ask for help with utmost sincerity, our whole being becomes a lightning rod, ready to be struck by rejuvenating lightning. This recovery is analogous to a doctor giving an electrical shock to someone whose heart has stopped beating. We can also be spiritually revived and set onto a new course of living.

The "death and resurrection show" (or ritual of rebirth) can happen over and over again. Each time we sit down on the bench to perform seiki jutsu, we surrender our dilemmas to the natural movements and allow them to revive us. When we allow the hands of a shaker to give us a shake, we surrender to a greater power outside (but including) ourselves. And when we go to a religious setting and throw ourselves before the Creator, we are orienting ourselves toward awakening the deepest transformation of our souls.

Shaking medicine, and all art for that matter, should never be "practiced." If you practice playing music, you will sound like you are practicing when you perform. Always perform your art and your life. Life is not a rehearsal; it is the real thing. Whenever you hear people talk about their spiritual practice, say to yourself, "I do not practice; I perform my life." Shaking is a performance, and all the occasions that call it forth are living Life Force Theatres. They are creative settings for working the spirit and being played by the spirit.

Know that when the spirit is in you, the shake is also in you. When the shake is inside, you never have to worry about activating it. It comes forth when it is necessary and appropriate for it to manifest itself. Seasoned shakers, who have the shaking spirit permanently inside, find themselves surprised by the ecstatic vibrations. When they are tired and lie down to rest, high-frequency vibrations come on their heads, providing instantaneous renewal. If they enter a sacred place where the spirit resides, they feel it and they want to shake and shout. They become, over the years, more than lightning rods. They become the lightning itself. The bolts or arrows of electricity live within their bellies. They are ready to be activated at a second's notice. Shaking medicine, both the receiving of it and the carrying of it, is a walking and talking mysterious electrical light show.

The greatest gift I have ever received in my life was the spirited shake. I carry it with me wherever I go. It electrifies and illumines my life and that of others who are open to its transformative current. It is free of charge, though highly charged, to anyone who sincerely seeks it. People are not able to know why they are here, what they are supposed to do, or who they are unless they are deeply shaken and attuned to the guiding force. Yes, the force is around you, and it is waiting for you to fully realize that it can be within you, bringing forth all the meanings, directions, resources, and answers you seek.

Stop trying to run away from your ignorance and your shortcomings. They are the entry ticket to getting leveled to the ground, enabling you, in turn, to be hit by lightning. And believe me, you will jump and jerk when the spiritual bolt hits you. When you experience its heightened arousal, you will thirst and hunger for its ongoing presence. You will be unable to stop pursuing a relationship with it.

At first, you will definitely want its spirit upon you, but if you surrender to a faith that reorders the priorities of your life, making you want to praise and honor the unnameable mystery that created you, a great miracle will take place. The spirited shake will enter and live inside you. You will become a shaking, spirited presence: a lighthouse and power supply station for others. If you want to see the light, you have to find the current that turns it on. Shaking medicine delivers all the juice needed to turn on the light and to turn on your life. Start jumping right now, knowing that this possibility of transformation is immediately present for you. The simple realization of this possibility is enough for you to bring forth a trembling of delight and expectation.

As I was growing up, I played the piano in the revival services of my father's church. At the end of each service, following all the teaching about the power of the Holy Spirit and how it can transform each person's life, a hymn was sung called a "hymn of invitation." As its words were sung, with lyrics such as "Come home, come home," the members of the congregation would be invited to open their hearts and become available to feel the "pulling" or "calling" of the spirit. If they felt it calling and pulling them, they were asked to come to the front of the church, announcing that they had felt the spirit and were surrendering their lives to it. It was the most emotional time in our church services, and my grandfather and father were masters at "bringing in the sheaves."

I would like to ask you to open your heart and be available for the spirit of life, however you define it, to touch you. Say to yourself, "I want to have spirit enter my life so that it may reside within me." Say that you are willing to get on the ground and fully humble yourself to the realization that when compared to the wisdom of the collective unconscious and the ecology of mind that pervades the planet Earth, you are an ignorant fool, incapable of directing your life toward fulfilling its destiny. Ask the spirit to enter and take over. Even if you have done this before, ask again. Ask the spirit to reenter your life with an even greater presence than you have ever known.

As it has for millions of people before you, spirit's first presence will feel like a gentle tugging and pulling. It may even tap your shoulder or whisper in your ear with the sound of wind, or a silent voice may calmly and surely call you. Allow the vibration to send a spiritual tremor inside you. It is the first lightning bolt. Consider accepting this calling, pulling, and trembling, so that you walk toward the mysteries that wait. Walk toward the kingdom of shaking wonders. Jump and shout with joy when you allow yourself to feel the enchantment of this very moment.

In closing, I offer a shaking ceremony for you to perform. The moment you feel a "tugging" or "pulling" or "calling" to shake, run to this book, immediately turn to this page, and follow these instructions:

Hold this book, *Shaking Medicine,* in your hand and shake it. Do so vigorously, pretending that the book will become highly charged by your motions. Consider that in an imaginary realm, the color of the ink of each word inside this book will change as it is energized and heated up. Don't open the book, but imagine that the shaking is changing the color of all the words and sentences. They move from being black, to being red, then blue, and finally become white. After shaking it through these colors, know that if you were to open the book, it would appear blank, as total whiteness. Nevertheless, you would know that the words are there, typed in white upon a white background. Call these the transformed words, the words that have been shaken into being inseparable from the universe that holds them.

As you stand shaking the book, have someone read these words to you:

"It is now time for you to shake everything that is essential about and within you. As you tremble and shake, imagine that all your ideas, feelings, hopes, and aspirations, along with their opposites, are being shaken. A great mixing and stirring and reorganization is being set in motion. You may begin to wonder whether everything that you have learned and everything that has happened to you has simply happened so that someday you'd have something to shake up. You cannot become who you were born to be unless all the parts are shaken into place. Consider believing this and acting upon it."

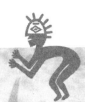

AFTERWORD

The First People Speak about
Shaking Medicine

The Juǀ'hoan Bushman *nǀom-kxaosi* (shamans) are the world's most experienced shakers, whose culture embodies the oldest form of healing on Earth. They are delighted that more of the world will know about shaking medicine, and they have asked for the opportunity to pronounce and clarify their own way of healing and ecstatic religion. The following declaration of the nǀom-kxaosi summarizes their understanding and practice of shaking medicine. These words were recorded, written, and approved for publication in September 2006 at Tsumkwe, Namibia.

DECLARATION OF THE NǀOM-KXAOSI
by ǀKunta Boo, N!yae Kxao, Tcoqa ǀUi, N!ae G≠kau,
Ti!'ae ≠Oma, Kxao Boo, ≠Oma Dahm, ǀXoan ǀChuǀkun, ǀui N!a'an, and
Gǀao'o Kaqece with Beesa Boo and Bradford Keeney

Anything spoken or written about our most important beliefs and healing ways must emphasize and reemphasize the importance of love, the Sky God, and the rising of our hearts. As our heartfelt feelings rise through loving God, we shake and step into the ability to heal others, as well as prepare to receive sacred lessons and gifts from the gods and ancestors.

If this kind of divine love isn't addressed more than anything else when someone talks about our ways, then that person simply does not know what he or she is talking about.

Many outsiders, especially anthropologists, have visited us over the years, and we have been very happy to welcome them. Some have become our close friends. However, there have been numerous misunderstandings and erroneous words, ideas, and theories published about our religious and healing ways. This declaration sets forth our statement about what it means to be a n l om-kxao, an owner (or master) of shaking medicine *(n l om)*.

Over the years, we have known and danced with Bradford Keeney. He has experienced what we experience and know about healing. He is a n l om-kxao and a *G≠aqba-n!a'an* ("Heart of the Spears") whose power is equal to ours. We give him the authority to speak on our behalf. He knows our truth because he experiences it. He is one of us.

We trust the translation and spellings of Beesa Boo, who is a leading translator of the Ju l 'hoan language into English. He has been a schoolteacher, a consultant in the correction of our dictionary, and has worked as an interpreter and translator for many anthropologists. He is fully aware of the misconceptions that have been portrayed by other writers. He accepts the responsibility for accurately telling our truth.

We, the n l om-kxaosi, affirm as strongly as we can that it is not our nature to lie about religious and healing knowledge. There are many things we have not spoken about to outsiders until the last decade. Most of our past responses to questions about healing were partial answers, because we felt the interviewer would not be able to understand our experience and way of knowing. Now it is urgent that we tell the whole story so that previous misunderstandings can be corrected. Most importantly, the world desperately needs what we know about God, love, and how we heal through shaking. We are the oldest culture on Earth, and we hold the oldest way of communicating with God. In these troubled times, our knowledge and wisdom are vitally important.

The knowledge and experiences of the Ju l 'hoan Bushman n l om-kxaosi, while having a common ground of understanding, allow room for individual differences. Our way of thinking is not illogical or problematically ambiguous, though it may appear that way to others. This is because we experience and know the world in a different way. In the old days, we called ourselves the people of the circle *(≠ahmi)*. We see everything in life as similar to the image of a dog chasing its tail. And we have referred to outsiders as straight-line people *(!hui juasi)*. We have always been aware of how difficult it is for outsiders to understand us. Now we are ready to make a new effort to teach those who care about how we live. These words are dedicated to the future generations of the Ju|'hoan and to all those whose hearts are open to shaking medicine.

In the beginning, before any time or place, there was the original force called N!o'an-kal'ae. It is the force that changes everything into good or bad. In the First Creation (≠Ain-≠aing≠ani), the original ancestors (G||auan≠'angsi) had a father (G≠koo N!a'an) and mother (Gauh-!o). The father and mother gave birth to creatures that kept changing into different animals. Among these creatures were the eland-headed people (N!ang-n|ais) who had hooves that made the sound of clapping. They became the first dancing n|om-kxaosi. There were various kinds of animal-headed people, and none of them ever became sick or died in First Creation.

The force that changes everything is behind the creation of all things, including the Sky God (!Xon!a'an). Anything created must change over and over again. This is the nature of First Creation. Even the Sky God, who lives in the eastern sky, has changing forms, each available for only a moment and quickly replaced by another form, behavior, feeling, and purpose. The changing forms are the way Trickster (|Xuri Kxaosi), who lives in the western sky, is revealed.

In Second Creation (G!xoa), when the animals were named, called "the great turning around" or Manisi n!a'an-na'an, the people and animals became separated from one another. The changing forms stopped changing because everything was given a stable name. Second Creation did not mean the end of First Creation. In a way, Second Creation is another example of the changing force of First Creation; this time, the whole changing world was changed into a non-changing world. N!o'an-kal'ae is still present today, and can interpenetrate Second Creation through the entry of the trickster forms of God. In Second Creation, people and animals get sick and die. To restore health and to ensure good relations, First Creation must breathe change and transformation into Second Creation.

The n|om-kxao's shaking (what we call *thara*) is a way of moving back and forth between First and Second Creation. This movement is the breathing and heartbeat of the creator Sky God and its never-ending creating. This is the pulse or vibration of n|om that raises our hearts and gives us renewed life. What we know about healing comes from the love we feel for and from the great Sky God.

There is no simple way to say what n|om is and what it isn't. But we all agree that its source is the Sky God's love. N|om is inseparable from music because songs make our hearts rise. The songs that have n|om are associated with the things we love, like water, honey, ostrich eggs, giraffes, elands, gemsbok, and so forth. The way n|om enters our bodies is through the needles *(||Auhsi)* and arrows *(≠oah tchiasi)* that are put into our g||abesi (belly and abdominal region) or into the top of our head *(||hang n!ang)*. If the g||abesi is "soft" *(g||abesi soan,* as we say), a needle or arrow of n|om may enter.

When the n|om comes straight from the Sky God or from the G!oah plant (a small bush), we call it a needle. When the n|om comes from an animal, such as a giraffe, eland, or oryx, among others, it is called an arrow *(tchiasi)*. The old words for needles used by our grandparents included *n!aihsi* and *||auh*. They often referred to them as "thorns" rather than needles.

The entry of a clean needle or arrow typically brings pain like that of a severe cramp or stinging tightness. The needles and arrows (referred to as needles henceforth) must be lined up correctly in the body (horizontally rather than vertically). They rest near the side or back of our g||abesi, and when they wake up, they move to the front of our belly.

The needles wake up when we sing and dance in a strong way. Our word for this kind of "waking up" is *!aia*. This word has been misunderstood by outsiders and regarded as *trance,* which is more akin to the daydreaming state you enter before falling asleep. !Aia is the opposite—it is more like the arousal and waking up you have when you wake up from sleep. However, what "wake up" in !aia are intense feelings. We define !aia as "waking up your strongest feelings and becoming reborn."

We also want to make clear that !aia does not have any meaning associated with death. Some anthropologists may have confused the word *!aia* with the word *!ai,* which means "real death." !Aia, the waking up of intense feelings, is stepping into your true self. To fully awaken !aia requires filling your heart with overwhelming love. As this happens, you move from seeing through your eyeballs to seeing through your feelings (*kxae ≠xaiai,* meaning "seeing the feeling"). As some of us say, the hot needles must rise from the g‖abesi to the heart, while the eyes must drop to the heart. !Aia is the movement of all our experience toward being inside the feelings of a fully loving heart.

The first moment of !aia is called *gaqm.* This is comparable to the moment when you strike a match to light a fire. It is the initial spark of waking up one's strong feelings, and it is the beginning of feeling a special sense of power. The first moments of being awakened are called *gua,* meaning "he or she has been lit." In a dance, the fire on the ground helps heat our inner power or inner fire *(n‖om-da'a).* The first station of !aia is called *n!aroh-‖xam,* in which fire is the dominating source of power. At this station of the dance, we feel power and self-importance. We may be tempted to show off and run into the fire, even placing our head into the flames. It is a place where fear is felt and faced. The first station is where beginners learn to wake up their needles and feel the cooked n‖om in their bodies. Here, you are a beginning owner of n‖om and are called a n‖om-kxao.

The next stage involves healing. It requires moving from raw power (a place of ignorance we call !Xaua-khoe) to a place of love. We call this the rising of our heart *(!ka tsau l'an).* The second phase is a stronger entry into !aia, and refers to entering the power of the heart rather than the power of the fire. In the beginning stage of a n‖om-kxao's development, inexperienced owners of n‖om are likely to show off and boast about their power. These people are called *n≠u'uhan-kxaosi.* They may also pretend that they are able to heal *(≠u'uhan)*. This second station, *g!a'ama-n!ausi,* is when the needles (and power) are lifted to the heart. Here our feelings are so strong that we feel great compassion for those who are sick. Fear is replaced by love. This is where we are able to heal and pull out sickness.

The strongest !aia takes us into the third stage or station, called *thara n⎮om*. This is when we most strongly tremble and shake. Here proper seeing—seeing through your feelings—is fully present. Thara (shaking) is not separate from !aia, as some writers have reported, and it is not limited to women. Thara is strong !aia, when our strong feelings make us shake. Thara n⎮om is the strongest and most meaningful shaking that enables us to give needles to others (l'*ua-n⎮om* means giving a needle to another person). In the final station, thara n⎮om, the needles are so hot that the n⎮om-kxao can give them to another person who is ready to receive them. At this stage of !aia, we feel inseparable from the gods and ancestors who are with(in) us.

A beginning n⎮om-kxao (a beginning learner is called a *n!aroh-ma*) does not necessarily know how to heal and remove sickness. He or she stays at the first station of the dance. Healing requires learning how to let the needles get extremely hot in the belly, resulting in a pulling motion in the abdomen. Here, we breathe heavily and shake mightily, and !aia deepens so that we have the strongest possible feeling of love for others at the dance. Our heart and g⎮⎮abesi feel as if they are going to burst. To get this strong, you must sing the songs in a powerful way, with your voice vibrating and further lifting your heart. When the needles are so hot that they turn to steam, they go out through the top of the head and fall to the ground, where they are cooled and turned back into needles that enter the bottom of the feet and are again recycled through the shaking body.

When we feel like this, we place our hands on a sick person and pull out the sickness *(≠hoe* is the word for pulling out the sickness with your hands and body). We must pull (use strong abdominal contractions) with the greatest desire to help the sick person. If we don't feel or pull hard enough, the sickness can get stuck inside us and make us sick. We must pull hard enough to release the sickness. We shout a cry, called

!'huhn, to give us the extra push we need to take out the sickness. The sound we make sounds like *kau-hariri.* The sickness may be dispelled from the n|om-kxao's body through an invisible hole in the back of the neck, called the *!ain-!'u,* or dispensed by shaking one's hands or exercising a "throwing away" motion.

There is some confusion among anthropologists about the nature of sickness and what role the deceased relatives, the ancestral *g||auansi,* play in sickness and healing. The needles inside us get dirty when bad feelings come toward us. Whenever a living or deceased person throws bad feelings at another, the recipient's needles get dirty. Sickness is caused by bad feelings. The worst of these feelings is anger, followed by jealousy and selfishness, among others. Again, these bad feelings may come from those who are living or those who are dead. A needle of sickness caused by the bad feelings of an ancestral spirit is called a *g||auansi tchi.*

When you see properly, you are able to see feelings. Bad feelings reveal themselves to the healer and require removal. If people have too many bad feelings while they are alive, they will continue to send dirty needles by their bad feelings when they become g||auansi. If you keep your needles clean while you are alive, then you will be able to help the living when you are a *g||auan.*

Bad feelings look very ugly (and are usually short), as a demon or a monster looks. They look different to each n|om-kxao, but they always look and smell bad. Good feelings look nice and have a good smell. Before a dance starts, even before you have deeply entered !aia, you might feel that there are some g||auansi around with bad feelings. That's when you can yell at them to go away and stop bothering the people. But as soon as you get strong and enter thara, the g||auansi's bad feelings run away. They are scared of the power of love.

The g||auansi with good feelings and love help us heal. We ask them not only to help us heal, but to teach us more things about healing as well. All strong dances attract the good g||auansi, and after such a dance we say to each other, "The ancestors were at the dance, and they were happy with our singing and dancing."

We want everyone to know that sickness and healing are not battles with the g‖auansi who want to make us sick. Healing is a cleansing of the dirt on our needles caused by bad feelings, whether thrown by the living or by the ancestral g‖auansi. We clean the dirty needles (and bad feelings) by the boiling power of love. Through raising the needles to our hearts, our bodies are able to heal others. When a n‖om-kxao is able to do this, he or she is called a *!aaiha*.

Many people have heard that the n‖om-kxaosi are able to turn themselves into animals, particularly lions. We call this shape-shifting process *thuru*. As a n‖om-kxao's needles get hot in station one (the power of the fire) and begin to move to station two (the power of love), there appears a side thread or rope that allows him or her to travel like an animal. The thread for lion thuru is called *tso*. Here, we feel as though we are lions, and along this thread our soul (not our body) can move about the land, seeing and hearing and feeling like a lion. The strongest n‖om-kxaosi avoid taking the threads of thuru, and instead raise the needles to their hearts, enabling the n‖om-kxaosi to move from raw power to pure love.

To a n‖om-kxao, the world can look like it is covered with a spider's web. These are the threads that connect everything and allow a n‖om-kxao to travel out of the body. The threads that all spirits, good and bad, travel on are called *maq*. Some of the threads are not good—they are dangerous and belong to the trickster. The red horizontal threads, for example, should be avoided. The best thread, felt and seen only by a n‖om-kxao whose heart has fully risen, is the thread or rope to the Sky God. This thread, called *!hui*, is vertical and takes one to the village in the sky. In this village, there is a special camelthorn tree *(n≠ahn)* that is seen by strong n‖om-kxao.

All vertical ropes and threads are capable of bending when you climb them. This turns a rope into a bad rope and returns you to emphasizing power rather than love. As we often say, "Trickster always has a fire trying to pull you toward it." The n‖om must remain strong to allow someone to climb straight up (or down). Strong vibrant singing and dancing by the n‖om-kxao and the community helps maintain the strength of the ropes so they won't bend and cause potential harm. The women's clapping must be strong enough to lift the dancers' feet, what we call *gu-tsau*.

There is no real distinction among threads, arrows, needles, songs, and nǀom, though we say that nǀom travels along the threads as an arrow that has been empowered (heated) by a song. The songs are the threads, and are the most important thing for a nǀom-kxao. The greatest gift one can receive from the gods and ancestors is ownership of a song. The nǀom songs awaken our strongest feelings, raise our hearts, and bring on the shaking that heals and provides entry to the gods and ancestors.

The most powerful nǀom is God's love, followed by our love for one another, love for the animals, and love for the plants. When you have ownership of something, it means that you own the feeling of love for it. This can be said only when a song is given that captures the feeling of that relationship and connection. The earliest nǀom song was probably the grass song and dance, which is like the G!oah women's dance that is popular today. Later, when the anthropologists and outsiders arrived in the 1950s, we were dancing to the eland and honey songs. When Beh ǁAo, a nǀom-kxao from Nǂaqmgoha, received the giraffe song, the giraffe dance was introduced by her husband, ǀAi!ae ǀUi, who was also a strong nǀom-kxao. Beh had been walking in the bush with some other women when several giraffes went running by them. In that moment, she caught the feeling of the giraffe and began moving and bobbing like it. She continued this movement on her way back to the village. That night, in a visionary dream, the giraffe song was given to her.

If someone asks for nǀom, we do not necessarily give it. We might say things such as, "If I give you nǀom, I'll be arrested and thrown in jail." Or we might try to push away the person by teasing with statements such as, "Nǀom will kill you. Why do you want to die?" The people who receive nǀom usually don't ask for it in a direct manner. They dance and sing strongly. When we see that their hearts are open in a good way, we will feel their gǁabesi and see if it is soft enough to receive a needle.

Some of the things written about our dance and healing practice are the things we say to those people who don't own nǀom or who are just beginning to learn. Please know that only beginning nǀom-kxaosi have great fear and are scared that they will die in the dance. The strongest n l om-kxaosi do not have fear and do not think they will die. They have moved from fear to love and to being instruments of the gods and ancestors. At this stage, they feel no pain. Receiving a needle "feels like being touched by water."

Death has nothing to do with the experience of a strong n l om-kxao. We only talk about "dying" in relationship to the dance in three ways: (1) an inexperienced n l om-kxao may be overwhelmed by intense feelings (!aia) in the dance and fall to the ground, losing consciousness. That is a dangerous time when the soul will leave the body. The strong n l om-kxaosi must go to this person and bring back the soul and restore life. This is not a good thing to happen. Strong n l om-kxaosi do not fall like this (with some exceptions) and falling has nothing to do with healing. (2) The second use of the conepts of *death* and *dying* is when a n l om-kxao has experienced a strong and long-lasting thara and says, "The needles have killed me." This means that the shaking has physically worn out that person. (3) Finally, the experienced n l om-kxaosi tease community members who either are not owners of n l om or are beginners, saying, "They will die if they are given a needle."

!Aaiha are not the strongest n l om-kxaosi. They are simply those who can pull out the sickness. The next level of n l om-kxaosi is called a *tco-kxao,* someone whose thara is so strong and developed that he or she can give needles to a person aspiring to be a n l om-kxao (or to another n l om-kxao who wants more needles). A person cannot decide to be a n l om-kxao, !aaiha, or tco-kxao. This is the Sky God's decision.

The strong n l om-kxaosi who also give the needles, the tco-kxaosi, are familiar with the three most powerful ecstatic experiences available to those who have been fully cooked: (1) climbing the threads to the sky village where the gods and ancestors reside—this climbing is called *n!uan-tso;* (2) receiving the Sky God's medicine water, called G!uaon l omga; and (3) the experience of union when two *n l om-kxaosi* shake together in the most powerful way—called Djxani-!uhsi. One way of doing this is for one person's heart to shake n l om into the other person's heart while they embrace. This way of transferring n l om is called ǂara-khoe.

As the needles cook and the n l om-kxao enters thara, no particular visual images are given importance. The focus is entirely on intense feelings that, in turn, create internal images seen by the mind. One's physical eyes are turned over to the eyes of the heart. We are not in a simple trance state, nor do we see any simple lines, dots, or wiggly shapes that change into human bodies with animal heads. We do not have that kind of experience. That idea comes from someone who is incorrectly guessing and does not know what we experience.

As we get stronger in the dance, our physical eyes see only a whirling world in which the fire often looks tall. We believe that the whirling is how First Creation looks. When we see First Creation as a whirling in the dance, we say that we see *!kabi*. We must learn to look past these images and focus solely on the seeing brought about by intense feeling.

We usually see and hear the gods and ancestors when we are sleeping. We call a visitation or sacred vision a *kabi*. It is regarded as distinct from dreams, which we call *!'un*. Most dreams are not important, though there are a few exceptions, such as when the ancestors make us dream about another person. A kabi is a visitation that we also refer to as "going to class." This is when we learn from the gods and ancestors. They teach us songs, dances, and other things.

They also may present you with gifts called !Xo tci. These might include an eland tail (N!ang !xui) or a dancing stick (!'hana) to use in the dance (to give needles by pointing at someone). Or one can receive a decorative ostrich feather (kxao-kxao! kui) or special skirt (!Oo) to wear in the dance. Men may receive a tortoise shell that holds medicine for heating up needles (Xuru a o n|om ga), while women may receive a tortoise shell that holds medicine for cooling down the needles (||'oara). Another gift is a hat from God that makes you strong when it is placed on your head. The hat is called Tci-n|oa ||ah jan.

Women n|om-kxaosi can have a kabi in which the Mother God teaches them about being a mother, or an ancestor may show them a necklace, bracelet, or skirt. These are gifts they present to us, and then we make them as we saw them in the kabi. When we have a kabi and actually see an ancestor or god, it is called a *cunkuri*. If we receive needles in a kabi, it is called *!'an-jukonaqnisi*.

The most important kabi involves receiving a song from the gods and ancestors. For example, prior to the introduction of the giraffe dance, the most important n ǀ om song and dance was the bee dance. One of its owners, Dham, grandfather of ≠oma Dham, had a kabi in which he saw a yellow flower burst open and become surrounded with large female bees as the ancestors sang in the background. He woke up singing the song, and the people gathered and celebrated the arrival of a new song and dance. We have different kinds of n ǀ om songs that we receive, including thara songs *(!aia tzisi)*, healing songs *(hoea khoe tzisi)*, prayer songs *(xom tzisi)*, and songs for communicating with the g ǁ auansi *(gaoan tzisi)*.

When we dance, we may remember what we have seen and heard in a kabi. This remembrance makes us have even stronger feelings, enhancing and intensifying our !aia. Those who have seen a thread to the sky village in a kabi will remember it in the dance. Their strong feelings about it will make them see it again with their feelings. In the same way, the ancestors can be felt and seen in the dance. They are seen through the heart's eyes, our truest eyes.

When a n ǀ om-kxao climbs a thread during a dance, he or she is remembering how it looked in a kabi while feeling its immediate presence. The feeling is so strong that the thread is re-seen by the heart's eyes. The intensity bends us over and we stomp while swinging our arms. As we feel ourselves climb, a guttural sound comes out of our mouths. The name of the sound made when climbing the thread is ǁxoan.

There are times when the n ǀ om is so hot, whether in the dance or in a kabi, that we will experience water pouring over the inside of our head and falling down within the rest of our body. Or we will receive a tortoise shell filled with liquid we can drink. This is God's medicine water.

The most powerful n ǀ om-kxaosi are called G≠aqba-n!a'an, which means "Heart of the Spears." They may know about the Sky God's special ostrich egg (!Xo dsuu-n!o), which holds the needles, threads, songs, and dances. Some G≠aqba-n!a'an have seen this ostrich egg in a kabi and have been reborn in it. The strongest n ǀ om-kxaosi receive a thread to the Sky God, called a !hui, when this ostrich egg is cracked open in a kabi. The G≠aqba-n!a'an feel less pain (or no pain) in the dance than other n|om-kxaosi. They live for awakening and experiencing the ecstatic gifts of n|om. They are often in thara, sometimes during the day and in their sleep at night. These n|om-kxaosi are referred to as "fully cooked by God." All n|om-kxaosi are depicted as thrown into God's pot (called *kaoha-kxo*). When you are fully cooked, God throws you out of the pot, and at that point you are regarded as a Heart of the Spears.

A fully cooked n|om-kxao has let go of all fear and has been smeared with a protective powder *(n≠hang)* by the Sky God. To pass through fear, a n|om-kxao has numerous kabi experiences that make him or her strong. For instance, a kabi may involve the n|om-kxao being sent (via vision) to the bottom of a water hole. As the n|om-kxao goes deeper into the water, it gets darker and requires courage to go all the way down to the bottom. Successful completion of this journey empowers the n|om-kxao and provides strength against all fear.

Only the G≠aqba-n!a'an are able to hold many different kinds of needles, songs, and n|om. For others, different kinds of n|om needles may compete and cause internal conflict. Some animal needles like those of the elephant (N!ang tchisi) don't mix well with G!oah plant needles (G!oahnaqnisi) or giraffe needles (≠Oah tchisi). However, the strongest n|om-kxaosi can hold all the different kinds of needles and arrows because these n|om-kxaosi are fully cooked. When a n|om-kxao has only one kind of n|om, it is described as singular—*n|om-tzi*. If a n|om-kxao has several kinds of n|om, it is described as plural—*n|om-tzisi*.

Some outsiders have said that a strong n|om-kxao is someone whom others want to have sex with. We want people to know that this is a mistake. Perhaps these writers were being teased by those they interviewed, or were talking with a n|om-kxao who wasn't on a good thread and was being influenced by Trickster. Or perhaps the writer was mentally disturbed. The truth is that we aim to raise the hot needles from our bellies to our hearts. When the heart rises, we do not feel sexuality. We go past that feeling. Instead, we feel love for everyone and a powerful desire to help those who are sick and suffering.

We also want people to know that there is as much healing with the women in their G!oah dance as there is with the men. Most of the strongest nǀom-kxaosi say that women are often the strongest healers because they are less tempted by power and find it easier to raise their hearts, the secret to all our spiritual and healing ways.

Our healing is about a love so strong that it makes you tremble and shake. When we dance the giraffe dance, we try to catch the feeling of the giraffe. When the giraffe needles (≠Oah tchisi) get hot enough, the thread *(tso)* between the giraffe and us gets stronger, enabling the giraffe's heart to enter our own hearts. We do not become the giraffe nor move about with it as we do in thuru. Here, we catch the feeling of the giraffe and dance for it. When this happens, the animal may show up the next day after the dance, making itself available for a hunt. Some strong male nǀom-kxaosi have had a special kabi in which they ride a giraffe, gemsbok, eland, or kudu. And they have made love to these animals in a kabi, "loving them in the same way they love their wives." This is the way it has always been for the Bushmen.

The Hearts of the Spears teach that everything must change in order to remain alive and well. We shake to experience the healing nǀom that moves back and forth between First and Second Creation. We shake because we feel God's love and are moved by it. We shake because it makes stronger the threads and ropes that connect all living things.

Our stories also shake. The old stories, which tell about First Creation, in which everything constantly changes, must be altered on each telling. The stories themselves shake and are capable of sending needles to the listeners. The key to understanding them is to be aware of how much change and transformation is instilled in their words and scenes. When a story mentions a body organ, it will typically emphasize the organ that embodies the most transformation (moving from one state to another). The best example is the intestine, the organ we regard as having the most nǀom. It is involved in the change from food to excrement. The nǀom-kxaosi desire to eat this organ because of its powerful nǀom. One owner of a giraffe song had a kabi in which the Sky God threw him into a giraffe's anus, and he ended up dancing in the animal's intestines.

Our bodies shake in the dance, and our stories shake when we tell them. Both activities can result in the transmission of needles. We also tremble and shake when we stand over the animal we have killed in a hunt. Hunting and gathering involve more than feeding ourselves. They are also ways to hunt and gather n|om. The way we share gifts and laugh and tease one another also helps the n|om flow. When we shake, we are made clean. This means that our feelings are centered on love and that we feel nothing bad toward anyone or anything.

Our grandparents called the threads *san||ae,* which means sinew. Through shaking love, the world and all of its relationships and interconnections are kept alive. We, the n|om-kxaosi, serve our gods and ancestors, keeping the sinews or threads of connection ready and available for all hearts to rise together and become one heart. Our most important concept is *!'oan,* which means the opening of your heart, and it is achieved through the most important feeling, the feeling of love, what we call *are.*

When the threads of relationship are strong, we feel the connections to all of life. When we need meat, the ancestors will pull a thread that is attached to an animal and to us. It will feel like a tapping on our body, called *≠a'am|'an.* We have many different kinds of tapping, all brought about by the threads of connection. The name for the tapping that means it is time for a hunt is *kxaetci!hun.* When a lion is near, we feel a shock on our fingertips called *!kau.* We feel a tapping in the palm of our hands when someone is about to give us a gift. And we feel tapping when friends and family are coming to visit us. A wife always feels a tapping between her legs in her vaginal area when her husband is returning from a hunt. Our bodies are attached to all the things we love, and these relationships are empowered by songs from the heart.

We often pray to the sky gods, who are our parents. The father is addressed as the Great Father, Mban!a'an. Throughout each day and night we simply pray, *!Xo hui mi,* which means "God help me." Our Great Mother, |aqn-|aqnce, is the Mother of the Bees. The bees are one of the greatest sources of n|om because they sing, dance, and make honey, which we love to eat. When you love the sky gods, you acquire a belief in them. This belief, brought about by the experience of love, is called *≠um !xo kokxui.*

There are times when we don't say the name of something that has a lot of n∣om. For example, when we are dancing, we won't utter the name of the dance or the songs or the needles. At that time, n∣om things are awakened and are too strong to even mention their names. Simply saying the name might result in getting a n∣om needle. We have other names that we can use, which we call "respect names." They enable us to name something without risking any attraction of its n∣om. For example, the respect name for n∣om is *tco*, whereas ≠*chisi* is the respect name for a giraffe n∣om arrow, and G≠kao Na'an is the respect name for the Sky God (!Xon!a'an).

When we die, the little g∣∣auansi children from long ago come to take our souls to the village in the sky. Our soul, *kxae ∣xoa,* is the living self with all its memories. It is part of our body when spirit, *n∣huin,* breathes through it. When we are alive on Earth, our soul is breathed out *(g!xa maq)* and then brought or breathed back *(n∣huin n'ang).* We must cultivate good feelings for each other now, so that we will be good to those we love when we become g∣∣auansi.

Our beliefs about religion and healing, called ≠*umsi !xo,* teach us that the Sky God lives in our heart, while the tricksters come into our mind. When our heart rises, it carries God's truth into our minds and gives us peace and joy. But when the voices of tricksters get into our head and fall to our heart, we find ourselves full of bad feelings, from jealousy to anger to selfishness. When people speak of God and do so primarily with a "head-filled heart," rather than a "heart-filled head," know that they speak for tricksters. Evil uses the words *good* and *God* to trick us into following a bad direction. Only trust the words of a love-filled heart that inspires true speech and thoughts. And above all things, aspire to be an "owner of God," *kxae ∣xoa,* which means that you own the feeling of love for God. This is the most important thing we have to teach. Its truth will deliver and nurture all other important truths.

NOTES

CHAPTER 1: THE SHAKE

1. Zane, *Journeys*, 100.

CHAPTER 2: THE CYCLE OF HEALING

1. D. Cohen, *The New Believers*, 101.
2. Gellhorn, "Further Studies," 69.
3. Quoted in Morgan, *T.T.T.*, 68.
4. Lex, "The Neurobiology of Ritual Trance."
5. Maturana and Varela, *The Tree of Knowledge.*
6. Von Foerster, *Cybernetics of Cybernetics.*
7. Quoted in Macnaughton, *Body, Breath & Consciousness*, 268.
8. Harner, *The Way of the Shaman*, 83.
9. Eliade, *The Sacred and the Profane*, 16.
10. Ibid., 24.
11. Ibid., 29.
12. Castagne, "Magie et Exorcism."
13. Eliade, *The Sacred and the Profane*, 100.
14. Quoted in Gore, *Ecstatic Body Postures*, ix.
15. Grof, *The Adventure of Self-Discovery*, 208–9.
16. Keeney, *Shaking Out the Spirits*, 1995.

CHAPTER 3: THE WORLD'S FIRST SHAKERS

1. Platvoet, *At War with God*, 2.
2. Keeney, *Ropes to God*, 142.

3. Keeney, *Bushman Shaman,* i.
4. Guenther, *Tricksters and Trancers,* 126.
5. Biesele, *Women Like Meat.*

CHAPTER 4: THE LAST TABOO

1. Fox, *The Spirit of Envy,* 11.
2. Ibid., 11.
3. Douglas, *George Fox.*
4. Janney, *History of the Religious Society of Friends,* 67.
5. Andrews, *The People Called Shakers,* 137.
6. Rose, "Prophesying Daughters," 97.
7. Mooney, "The Ghost Dance Religion," 239.
8. Quoted in Mooney, 940.
9. Barclay, *Inner Life,* 312.
10. Mavor and Dix, *Manitou.*
11. Quoted in Mooney, "The Ghost Dance Religion."
12. Haskett, *Shakerism Unmasked,* 144–46.
13. Mavor and Dix, *Manitou,* 197.
14. Andrews, *The People Called Shakers,* 137.
15. Sweet, *Religion of the American Fronter,* 10.
16. Blinn, *The Manifestation of Spiritualism,* 8.
17. Ibid., and Andrews, *The People Called Shakers.*
18. Andrews, *The People Called Shakers,* 158.
19. Poole, *Spiritualism.*
20. Lamson, *Two Years' Experience,* 2.
21. Blinn, *The Manifestation of Spiritualism,* 19–20.
22. Lamson, *Two Years' Experience,* 3.
23. Evans, *Shakers Compendium.*
24. Blinn, *The Manifestation of Spiritualism.*
25. Ibid., 22.
26. Quoted in Andrews, *The People Called Shakers.*
27. R. Emerson, "Goethe; or, the Writer," 1.

CHAPTER 5: EXPERIENCE VERSUS IDEOLOGY

1. Quoted in Deegan, *History of Mason County.*
2. Castile, "The 'Half-Catholic' Movement," 173.
3. Ober, "A New Religion," 592.
4. Gunther, "The Shaker Religion of the Northwest," 97.
5. Smith, "The Puyallup/Nisqually," 85.
6. Gould and Furukawa, "Aspects of Ceremonial Life," 55.
7. Quoted in Ruby and Brown, *John Slocum,* 39.
8. Waterman, "Paraphernalia," 553–54.

9. Hallowell, *The Role of Conjuring.*
10. Gunther, "The Shaker Religion of the Northwest," 100.
11. Quoted in Rakestraw, "The Quaker Indians of Puget Sound," 704.
12. Ober, "A New Religion," 585.
13. Amoss, *Coast Salish Dancing,* 136.
14. Mooney, "The Ghost Dance Religion," 746.
15. McLean, quoted in Mavor and Dix, *Manitou,* 366.
16. Mooney, "The Ghost Dance Religion," 783.
17. Ibid.
18. Olson, "The Quinault Indians," 173.
19. Klan, "The Shakers," 23.
20. Quoted in Ruby and Brown, *John Slocum,* 61.
21. Ober, "A New Religion," 588.
22. Quoted in Mooney, "The Ghost Dance Religion," 748.
23. Keeney, *Bushman Shaman.*
24. Keeney, *Guarani Shamans.*
25. Barnett, *A Messianic Cult,* 223.
26. Quoted in Ruby and Brown, *John Slocum,* 173–74.
27. Sackett, "The Siletz Indian Shaker Church," 124.
28. Mooney, "The Ghost Dance Religion," 754.
29. Ibid.
30. Pagels, *The Gnostic Gospels,* 13–14.
31. Ober, "A New Religion," 585.
32. Biesle, *Women Like Meat,* 73.

CHAPTER 6: HARNESSING THE SHAKE

1. Henney, "The Shakers of St. Vincent," 230.
2. Zane, *Journeys to the Spirit Lands,* 160.
3. Edric Commor quoted in Stephens, *The Spiritual Baptist Faith,* 18.
4. Keeney, *Shakers of St. Vincent.*
5. Ibid.
6. Stephens, *The Spiritual Baptist Faith,* 149.
7. Henney, "The Shakers of St. Vincent," 239.

CHAPTER 7: SINGING DOWN THE SPIRIT

1. Goreau, *Just Mahalia, Baby,* 55.
2. *The Apostolic Faith,* May 1907.
3. Ibid
4. Ibid.
5. Stuernagel, "Being Filled," 8.
6. Hurston, "Ritualistic Expression."

7. Pitts, *Old Ship of Zion*, 94.
8. Thorpe, "Life in Virginia."
9. Work, *Folk Song*, 38.
10. Ibid., 151.
11. J. Johnson, *God's Trombones*, 13.
12. Quoted in Willett, "Voices Raised," 3.
13. Sobel, *Trabelin' On*, 143.
14. Ibid., 145.
15. Pitts, *Old Ship of Zion*, 59.
16. C. Johnson, *God Struck Me Dead*.
17. Thompson, "The Shakers and Indian Shakers," 109.
18. Ibid., 63.
19. Ibid., 147.
20. Hurston, *The Sanctified Church*, 85.
21. C. Johnson, *God Struck Me Dead*, 44–45.
22. Hurston, *The Sanctified Church*, 90.
23. Hinson, *Fire in My Bones*, 2.
24. Ibid., 68.

CHAPTER 9: COILED WISDOM

1. Krishna, *Kundalini*, 186.
2. Sansonese, *The Body of Myth*, 245.
3. D. Johnson, *Body, Spirit, and Democracy*, 8.
4. Maitland, *Spacious Body*, 86.
5. Mookerjee and Kanna, *The Tantric Way*.
6. Waters, *Book of the Hopi*, 9.
7. Campbell, *The Inner Reaches*, 83.
8. Yogananda, *Autobiography of a Yogi*, 169.
9. Snyder, *The Practice of the Wild*, 102.
10. Kalweit, *Shamans, Healers, and Medicine Men*, 231.
11. Quoted in van Dusen, *The Presence of Other Worlds*, 49.
12. Whitman, preface to *Leaves of Grass*.

CHAPTER 10: THE LIFE FORCE THEATRE

1. Fulford, *Dr. Fulford's Touch of Life*, ix.
2. K. Cohen, *The Way of Qigong*, 372.

CHAPTER 11: THE ULTIMATE MEDICINE

1. Quoted in Mack, *Visionary Women*, 220.

BIBLIOGRAPHY

Akstein, David. *Teste do Reflexo Concentrador.* Campinos: Editora PSY, 1998.
———. *Un Voyage a Travers la Transe: La Terpsichore TranseTherapie.* Paris: Editions Sand, 1992.
Amoss, Pamela. *Coast Salish Dancing: The Survival of an Ancestral Religion.* Seattle: University of Washington Press, 1978.
Andrews, Edward Deming. *The People Called Shakers: A Search for the Perfect Society.* Oxford: Oxford University Press, 1953.
The Apostolic Faith 1, no. 8 (May 1907).
Avalon, Arthur. *The Serpent Power.* New York: Dover, 1974.
Barclay, Robert. *Inner Life of Religious Societies of the Commonwealth.* London: Hodder & Sloughton, 1876.
Barnett, H. G. *Indian Shakers: A Messianic Cult of the Pacific Northwest.* Carbondale: Southern Illinois University Press, 1972.
Bateson, Gregory. *Mind and Nature: A Necessary Unity.* New York: E. P. Dutton, 1979.
———. "Some Components of Socialization for Trance." *Ethos* 3 (1975): 144–55.
———. *Steps to an Ecology of Mind.* New York: Ballantine Books, 1972.
Becker, Robert O. *The Body Electric: Electromagnetism and the Foundation of Life.* New York: Morrow, 1985.
Bell, Hesketh J. *Obeah: Witchcraft in the West Indies.* Westport, Conn.: Negro Universities Press, 1970.
Belo, Jane. *Trance in Bali.* New York: Columbia University Press, 1960.
Benson, Herbert. *Beyond the Relaxation Response: How to Harness the Healing Power of Your Personal Beliefs.* New York: Berkley Books, 1984.
———. *The Relaxation Response.* New York: Morrow, 1975.

————. *Timeless Healing: The Power and Biology of Belief.* New York: Fireside, 1997.

Bentov, Itzhak. *Stalking the Wild Pendulum.* Rochester, Vt.: Destiny Books, 1988.

Berggren, Karen. *Circle of Shaman: Healing Through Ecstasy, Rhythm, and Myth.* Rochester, Vt.: Destiny Books, 1998.

Biesele, Megan. *Women Like Meat: The Folklore and Foraging Ideology of the Kalahari Ju|'hoansi.* Johannesburg: Witwatersrand University Press, 1993.

Bleek, W. H. I., and L. C. Lloyd. *Specimens of Bushmen Folklore.* London: George Allen & Co. Ltd., 1911.

Bleek, D. F., ed. "Beliefs and Customs of the |Xam Bushmen." *Bantu Studies* 9 (1935).

Blinn, Henry Clay. *The Manifestation of Spiritualism among the Shakers 1837–1847.* East Canterbury, N.H.: 1899.

Branch, Christian William. "The Endemic Religious Insanity of St. Vincent." *The Monist* 17 (1907): 299–310.

Bunyan, John. *The Pilgrim's Progress.* Oxford: Oxford University Press, 1984.

Burr, Harold Saxton. *Blueprint for Immortality: The Electric Patterns of Life.* Essex, England: C. W. Daniel, 1972.

Butler, Lee H., Jr. "The Evolution of Shamanism within the African American Christian Church." http://members.aol.com/sarjournal/issue5ar.htm, accessed 12/29/2000.

Campbell, Joseph. *The Inner Reaches of Outer Space.* New York: Harper Collins, 1986.

Casanowicz, I. M. "Shamanism of the Natives of Siberia." *Annual Report of the Smithsonian Institution.* Washington, D.C., 1926.

Castagne, J. "Magie et Exorcisme Chez les Kazak-Kirghizes et Autres Peoples Turcs Orientaux." *Revue des Études Islamiques* (1930): 53–151.

Castile, George P. "The 'Half-Catholic' Movement: Edwin and Myron Eells and the Rise of the Indian Shaker Church." *Pacific Northwest Quarterly* 73 (1982): 165–74.

Chalcraft, Edwin L. "The 'Shaker' Religion of the Indians of the Northwest." *The Assembly Herald* 19 (February 1913): 74–75.

Cleary, Thomas. *Vitality, Energy, Spirit.* Boston: Shambhala, 1992.

Cohen, Daniel. *The New Believers.* New York: M. Evans & Co., 1975.

Cohen, Kenneth S. *Honoring the Medicine.* New York: Ballantine Books, 2003.

————. *The Way of Qigong: The Art and Science of Chinese Energy Healing.* New York: Ballantine Books, 1997.

Crapanzano, Vincent, and Vivian Garrison, eds. *Case Studies in Spirit Possession.* New York: John Wiley and Sons, 1977.

Deegan, Harry W. *History of Mason County, Washington.* Shelton, Wash., 1971.

Douglas, Major. *George Fox: The Red Hot Quaker.* Cincinnati: Revivalist Press, n.d.

Duerr, Hans Peter. *Dreamtime: Concerning the Boundary Between Wilderness and Civilization.* Oxford: Basil Blackwell, 1985.

Eisenberg, David, with Thomas Lee Wright. *Encounters with Qi: Exploring Chinese Medicine.* New York: Bantam, 1989.

Eliade, Mircea. *The Sacred and the Profane: The Nature of Religion.* New York: Harvest Books, 1968.

Elkins, Hervey. *Fifteen Years in the Senior Order of Shakers: A Narration of Facts, Concerning That Singular People.* Hanover, N.H.: Dartmouth Press, 1853.

Emerson, V. F. "Can Belief Systems Influence Behavior? Some Implications of Research on Meditation." *Newsletter Review,* R. M. Bucke Memorial Society, vol. 5 (1972): 20–32.

Emerson, Ralph Waldo. "Goethe; or, The Writer." In *Representative Men: The Collected Works of Ralph Waldo Emerson,* volume 4. Cambridge: Harvard University Press, 1987.

Erickson, Betty Alice, and Bradford Keeney. *Milton H. Erickson, M.D.: An American Healer.* Philadelphia: Ringing Rocks Press, 2006.

Erickson, Milton H. *The Collected Papers of Milton H. Erickson.* Edited by Ernest S. Rossi. New York: Irvington, 1980.

Evans, F. W. *Shakers Compendium.* New York: D. Appleton & Co., 1859.

Fischer, Roland. "A Cartography of the Ecstatic and Meditative States." *Science* 174 (1971): 897–904.

Ford, Clyde W. *Where Healing Waters Meet: Touching Mind and Emotion Through the Body.* Barrytown, N.Y.: Station Hill Press, 1989.

Fox, George. *Autobiography.* London: Headly Bros., 1904.

———. *The Journal of George Fox.* Edited by John L. Nichols. Cambridge: Cambridge University Press, 1952.

———. *The Spirit of Envy, Lying, and Persecution, Made Manifest.* London, 1663.

Fulford, Robert C., with Gene Stone. *Dr. Fulford's Touch of Life: The Healing Power of the Natural Life Force.* New York: Pocket Books, 1996.

Garrett, Clarke. *Spirit Possession and Popular Religion: From the Camisards to the Shakers.* Baltimore: The Johns Hopkins University Press, 1987.

Gellhorn, E. "Further Studies on the Physiology and Pathophysiology of the Tuning of the Central Nervous System." *Psychosomatics* 10 (1969): 94–104.

Gerber, Richard. *Vibrational Medicine.* Santa Fe: Bear & Co., 1988.

Giri, Swami Satyeaswarananda. *Kriya: Finding the True Path.* San Diego: Sanskrit Classics, 1991.

———. *Kriya Sutras of Babaji.* San Diego: Sanskrit Classics, 1994.

Glazier, Stephen D. *Marchin' the Pilgrims Home: A Study of the Spiritual Baptists of Trinidad.* Salem, Wis.: Sheffield Publishing Company, 1993.

Goodman, Felicitas D. *Ecstasy, Ritual, and Alternate Reality: Religion in a Pluralistic World.* Bloomington: Indiana University Press, 1988.

————. *Where the Spirits Ride the Wind: Trance Journeys and Other Ecstatic Experiences.* Bloomington: Indiana University Press, 1990.

Gore, Belinda. *Ecstatic Body Postures: An Alternate Reality Workbook.* Santa Fe: Bear & Co., 1995.

Goreau, L. *Just Mahalia, Baby.* Waco, Tex.: World Books, 1975.

Gould, Richard A., and Theodore Paul Furukawa. "Aspects of Ceremonial Life Among the Indian Shakers of Smith River, California." *Kroeber Anthropological Papers* 31 (1962): 51–67.

Greenwell, Bonnie. *Energies of Transformation: A Guide to the Kundalini Process.* Valencia, Calif.: Delta Lithograph, 1988.

Grof, Stanislav. *The Adventure of Self-Discovery: Dimensions of Consciousness and New Perspectives in Psychotherapy and Inner Exploration.* Albany: State University of New York Press, 1988.

Grossing, Gerhard. "Comparing the Long-Term Evolution of 'Cognitive Invariance' in Physics with a Dynamics in States of Consciousness." *Foundations of Science* 6 (2001): 255–72.

Grossinger, Richard. *Planet Medicine: Modalities.* Berkeley, Calif.: North Atlantic, 1995.

Guenther, Mathias. *The Nharo Bushmen of Botswana: Tradition and Change.* Hamburg: Helmut Buske Verlag, 1986.

————. *Tricksters and Trancers.* Bloomington: Indiana University Press, 1999.

Gullick, Charles. "Shakers and Ecstasy." *New Fire* 9 (1971): 7–11.

Gunther, Erna. "The Shaker Religion of the Northwest." In *The Northwest Mosaic: Minority Conflicts in Pacific Northwest History,* edited by James A. Halseth and Bruce Glasrud, 85–102. Boulder, Colo.: Pruett Publishing Co., 1977.

Halifax, Joan. *Shaman: The Wounded Healer.* New York: Thames and Hudson, 1982.

————. *Shamanic Voices: A Survey of Visionary Narratives.* New York: E. P. Dutton, 1979.

Hallowell, A. Irving. *The Role of Conjuring in Salteaux Society.* Philadelphia: University of Pennsylvania Press, 1942.

Harmon, Ray. "Indian Shaker Church: The Dalles." *Oregon Historical Quarterly* 72 (1971): 148–58.

Harner, Michael. *The Way of the Shaman.* New York: Bantam, 1982.

Harpur, Tom. *The Uncommon Touch: An Investigation of Spiritual Healing.* Toronto: McClelland and Stewart, 1994.

Haskett, William J. *Shakerism Unmasked.* Pittsfield, Mass.:1828.

Havecker, Cyril. *Understanding Aboriginal Culture.* Sydney: Cosmos Periodicals, 1987.

Hazzard-Gordon, Katrina. "Dancing to Rebalance the Universe: African American Secular Dance and Spirituality." *Black Sacred Music* 7 (1993): 17–28.

Henney, Jeannette. "'Mourning': A Religious Ritual Among the Spiritual Baptists of St. Vincent: An Experience in Sensory Deprivation." Working Paper 21, Cross-Cultural Study of Dissociational States, 1968.

———. "The Shakers of St. Vincent: A Stable Religion." In *Religion, Altered States of Consciousness, and Social Change*, edited by Erika Bourguignon. Columbus: Ohio State University Press, 1973.

———. "Trance Behavior Among the Shakers of St. Vincent." Working Paper 8, Cross-Cultural Study of Dissociational States, April 1967.

Herrigel, Eugen. *Zen in the Art of Archery*. New York: Pantheon, 1953.

Herskovits, Melville J., and Frances S Herskovits. *Trinidad Village*. New York: Alfred A. Knopf, 1947.

Hinson, Glenn. *Fire in My Bones: Transcendence and the Holy Spirit in African American Gospel*. Philadelphia: University of Pennsylvania Press, 2000.

Holloway, Mark. *Heavens on Earth: Utopian Communities in America 1680–1880*. New York: Dover, 1966.

Horgan, Edward R. *The Shaker Holy Land: A Community Portrait*. Boston: The Harvard Common Press, 1982.

Houk, James T. *Spirits, Blood, and Drums: The Orisha Religion in Trinidad*. Philadelphia: Temple University Press, 1995.

Hunt, Valerie V. *Infinite Mind: The Science of Human Vibrations*. Malibu, Calif.: Malibu Publishing, 1995.

Hurston, Zora Neale. "Ritualistic Expression from the Lips of the Communicants of the Seventh Day Church of God, Beaufort, South Carolina." Library of Congress: Collections of the Manuscript Division, 1940.

———. *The Sanctified Church*. Berkeley, Calif.: Turtle Island, 1981.

Irving, Darrel. *Serpent of Fire: A Modern View of Kundalini*. York Beach, Maine: Samuel Weiser Inc., 1995.

Ishii, Jozo. *The Essentials of Self-Healing Therapy*. Japan, 1928.

Janney, S. M. *History of the Religious Society of Friends, From Its Rise to the Year 1828*. 4 vols. Philadelphia: T. E. Zell, 1859–67.

Jochelson, Waldemar I. "The Yukaghir and the Yukaghirized Tungus." In *Jesup North Pacific Expedition IX*, 2 vols. American Museum of Natural History Memoirs 13, 2–3 (1924–26).

Johnson, Clifton H. *God Struck Me Dead: Religious Conversion Experiences and Autobiographies of Ex-slaves*. Philadelphia: Pilgrim Press, 1969.

Johnson, Don Hanlon. *Body, Spirit, and Democracy*. Berkeley, Calif.: North Atlantic Books, 1994.

———. *Bone, Breath & Gesture*. Berkeley: North Atlantic Books, 1995.

Johnson, James Weldon. *God's Trombones: Seven Negro Sermons in Verse*. New York: The Viking Press, 1955.

Kalweit, Holger. *Shamans, Healers, and Medicine Men*. Boston: Shambhala, 1987.

Katz, Richard. *Boiling Energy: Community Healing Among the Kalahari !Kung.* Cambridge: Harvard University Press, 1982.

Katz, Richard, Megan Biesele, and Verna St. Denis. *Healing Makes Our Hearts Happy.* Rochester, Vt.: Inner Traditions, 1997.

Keeney, Bradford. *Aesthetics of Change.* New York: Guilford Press, 1983.

———. *Balians: Traditional Healers of Bali.* Philadelphia: Ringing Rocks Press, 2004.

———. *Brazilian Hands of Faith.* Philadelphia: Ringing Rocks Press, 2003.

———. *Bushman Shaman: Awakening the Spirit through Ecstatic Dance.* Rochester, Vt.: Destiny Books, 2005.

———. "Dancing with the Bushmen." *Spirituality and Health,* June 2003.

———. *The Energy Break.* New York: Golden Books, 1998.

———. *Everyday Soul.* New York: Riverhead, 1996.

———. *Gary Holy Bull: Lakota Yuwipi Man.* Philadelphia: Ringing Rocks Press, 1999.

———. *Guarani Shamans of the Rainforest.* Philadelphia: Ringing Rocks Press, 2000.

———. *Ikuko Osumi, Sensei: Japanese Master of Seiki Jutsu.* Philadelphia: Ringing Rocks Press, 1999.

———. *Kalahari Bushman Healers.* Philadelphia: Ringing Rocks Foundation, 1999.

———. *Ropes to God: Experiencing the Bushman Spiritual Universe.* Philadelphia: Ringing Rocks Press, 2003.

———. *Shakers of St. Vincent.* Philadelphia: Ringing Rocks Press, 2002.

———. *Shaking Out the Spirits.* New York: Station Hill Press, 1995.

———. *Shamanic Christianity: The Direct Experience of Mystical Communion.* Rochester, Vt.: Destiny Books, 2006.

———. *Vusamazulu Credo Mutwa: Zulu High Sanusi.* Philadelphia: Ringing Rocks Press, 2001.

———. *Walking Thunder: Dine Medicine Woman.* Philadelphia: Ringing Rocks Foundation, 2001.

Kerr, Hugh T., and John M. Mulder. *Famous Conversions.* Grand Rapids, Mich.: Wm. B. Eerdmans Pub. Co., 1983.

Klan, Yvonne. "The Shakers." *Raincoast Chronicles* 7 (1977): 20–24.

Kostarelos, Frances. *Feeling the Spirit: Faith and Hope in an Evangelical Black Storefront Church.* Columbia: University of South Carolina Press, 1995.

Kottler, Jeffrey, and Jon Carlson, with Bradford Keeney. *American Shaman: An Odyssey of Global Healing Traditions.* New York: Brunner-Routledge, 2004.

Krieger, Dolores. *Therapeutic Touch: How to Use Your Hands to Help or to Heal.* Englewood Cliffs, N.J.: Prentice-Hall, 1979.

Krippner, Stanley, and Patrick Welch. *Spiritual Dimensions of Healing: From Native Shamanism to Contemporary Health Care.* New York: Irvington, 1992.

Krishna, Gopi. *Kundalini: The Evolutionary Energy in Man*. Boston: Shambhala Publications, 1970.

———. *Living with Kundalini: The Autobiography of Gopi Krishna*. Boston: Shambhala Publications, 1993.

Kriyananda, Goswami. *The Kriya Yoga Upanishad and the Mystical Upanishads*. Chicago: Temple of Kriya Yoga, 1993.

Lamson, David. *Two Years' Experience Among the Shakers: Being a Description of the Manners and Customs of that People, the Nature and Policy of their Government, their Marvelous Intercourse with the Spiritual World, the Object and Uses of Confession, their Inquisition, in Short, a Condensed View of Shakerism as It Is*. West Boylston, Mass., 1848.

Larsen, Stephen. *The Shaman's Doorway: Opening Imagination to Power and Myth*. Rochester, Vt.: Inner Traditions, 1998.

Lawlor, Robert. *Voices of the First Day: Awakening in the Aboriginal Dreamtime*. Rochester, Vt.: Inner Traditions, 1991.

Levett, Carl. *Crossings: A Transpersonal Approach*. Boston: Branden Publishing Co., 1974.

Levine, Peter A., with Ann Frederick. *Waking the Tiger: Healing Trauma*. Berkeley, Calif.: North Atlantic Books, 1997.

Levy, Mark. *Technicians of Ecstasy: Shamanism and the Modern Artist*. Norfolk, Conn.: Bramble Books, 1993.

Lewis-Williams, David. *Images of Power: Understanding Bushmen Rock Art*. Johannesburg: Southern Book Publishers, 1989.

Lex, Barbara W. "The Neurobiology of Ritual Trance." In *The Spectrum of Ritual: A Biogenetic Structural Analysis,* edited by Eugene G. d'Aquili, Charles D. Laughlin Jr., and John McManus. New York: Columbia University Press, 1979.

Lober, Irene. *Auf eigenen Fussen gehen: Somato-psychologische Erfahrungen einer ehemals Querschnittsgelahmten*. Lohnrbach: Der Grune Zweig, 1989.

Lorca, Federico García. "Play and Theory of the Duende." In *Deep Song and Other Prose,* edited and translated by Christoher Mauere. New York: New Directions, 1975.

Lovelace, Earl. *The Wine of Astonishment*. Oxford: Heinemann, 1982.

Mack, Phyllis. *Visionary Women: Ecstatic Prophecy in Seventeenth Century England*. Berkeley: University of California Press, 1992.

Macnaughton, Ian. *Body, Breath & Consciousness: A Somatics Anthology*. Berkeley, Calif.: North Atlantic Books, 2004.

Maitland, Jeffrey. *Spacious Body: Explorations in Somatic Ontology*. Berkeley, Calif.: North Atlantic Books, 1995.

Maturana, Humberto R., and Francisco J. Varela. *The Tree of Knowledge: The Biological Roots of Human Understanding*. Boston: Shambhala, 1987.

Mavor, James W., Jr., and Byron E. Dix. *Manitou: The Sacred Landscape of New England's Native Civilization*. Rochester, Vt.: Inner Traditions, 1989.

McNemar, Richard. *The Kentucky Revival*. Cincinnati, 1807.

Miner, Malcolm. *Your Touch Can Heal: A Guide to Healing Touch and How to Use It.* Keswick, Va.: Faith Ridge, 1990.

Mischel, Frances O. "African Powers in Trinidad: The Shango Cult." *Anthropological Quarterly* 30 (1957): 45–59.

"A Missionary Family." *The Apostolic Faith* 1, no. 8 (May 1907): 2.

Mookerjee, Ajit. *Kundalini: The Arousal of the Inner Energy.* Rochester, Vt.: Destiny Books, 1991.

Mookerjee, Ajit, and Madhu Kanna. *The Tantric Way.* London: Thames and Hudson, 1977.

Mooney, James. "The Ghost Dance Religion." In *Fourteenth Annual Report of the Bureau of Ethnology to the Smithsonian Institution.* Washington, D.C.: Government Printing Office, 1892–93.

Morgan, Doug. *T.T.T.: An Introduction to Trance Dancing.* Lantzville, British Columbia: Ship Cottage Press, 1988.

Murphy, Joseph M. *Working the Spirit: Ceremonies of the African Diaspora.* Boston: Beacon Press, 1994.

Neumann, Erich. *The Origins and History of Consciousness.* New York: Pantheon Books, 1954.

Ni, Maoshing. *The Yellow Emperor's Classic of Medicine.* Boston: Shambhala, 1995.

Norbu, Thinley. *Magic Dance: The Display of the Self-Nature of the Five Wisdom Dakinis.* Boston: Shambhala, 1999.

Ober, Sarah Endicott. "A New Religion Among the West Coast Indians." *Overland Monthly* 56 (July–December 1910): 583–94.

Odier, Daniel. *Tantric Quest: An Encounter with Absolute Love.* Rochester, Vt.: Inner Traditions, 1997.

Olson, Roland. "The Quinault Indians." *University of Washington Publications in Anthropology* 6 (1936): 1–190.

Osumi, Ikuko, and Malcolm Ritchie. *The Shamanic Healer: The Healing World of Ikuko Osumi and the Traditional Art of Seiki Jutsu.* Rochester, Vt.: Healing Arts Press, 1988.

Otto, Rudolph. *The Idea of the Holy.* Translated by John W. Aarvey. New York: Oxford University Press, 1958.

Pagels, Elaine. *The Gnostic Gospels.* New York: Vintage, 1979.

Pitts, Walter. *Old Ship of Zion.* New York: Oxford University Press, 1993.

Platvoet, Jan G. "At War with God: Ju|'hoan Curing Dances." *Journal of Religion in Africa* 29 (1999): 2–62.

Pollack, Andrew. "The Life Force in the Briefcase." The *New York Times,* November 28, 1995, C1–C2.

Poole, Cyrus O. *Spiritualism as Organized by the Shakers.* Mt. Lebanon, N.Y., 1887.

Rakestraw, Charles D. "The Shaker Indians of Puget Sound." *The Southern Workman* 29 (1900): 702–709.

Reagan, Albert B. "The Shake Dance of the Quilente Indians, with Drawing by an Indian Pupil of the Quilente Day School." *Proceedings of the Indiana Academy of Science* (1908): 71–74.

A Return of Departed Spirits of the Highest Characters of Distinction, as Well as the Indiscriminate of All Nations, into the Bodies of the "Shakers" or "United Society of Believers in the Second Advent of the Messiah." Philadelphia: J. R. Cohen, 1843.

Ripinsky-Naxon, Michael. *The Nature of Shamanism: Substance and Function of a Religious Metaphor.* Albany: State University of New York Press, 1993.

Rose, Judith. "Prophesying Daughters: Testimony, Censorship, and Literacy Among Early Quaker Women. *Critical Survey* 14 (2002): 93–110.

Rouget, Gilbert. *Music and Trance: A Theory of the Relations between Music and Possession.* Chicago: The University of Chicago Press, 1985.

Ruby, Robert H. "A Healing Service in the Shaker Church." *Oregon Historical Society* 67 (1966): 347–55.

Ruby, Robert H., and John A. Brown. *John Slocum and the Indian Shaker Church.* Norman: University of Oklahoma Press, 1996.

Sackett, Lee. "The Siletz Indian Shaker Church." *Pacific Northwest Quarterly* 64 (1973): 120–26.

Sanders, Cheryl J. *Saints in Exile: The Holiness-Pentecostal Experience in African American Religion and Culture.* Oxford: Oxford University Press, 1996.

Sannella, Lee. *The Kundalini Experience.* Lower Lake, Calif.: Integral, 1987.

Sansonese, J. Nigro. *The Body of Myth: Mythology, Shamanic Trance, and the Sacred Geometry of the Body.* Rochester, Vt.: Inner Traditions, 1994.

Schwarz, Jack. *The Human Energy System.* New York: E. P. Dutton, 1980.

Shaffer, Carolyn. "An Interview with Emilie Conrad Da'Oud." *The Yoga Journal* 77 (1987): 52.

Shih, Tzu Kuo. *Qi Gong Therapy: The Chinese Art of Healing with Energy.* Barrytown, N.Y.: Station Hill, 1994.

Sieroszewski, Wenceslas. *Yakuty.* St. Petersburg: Tipografia Glavnogo Upravleniia Udelov, 1896.

Simpson, George E. "Baptismal, 'Mourning,' and 'Building': Ceremonies of the Shouters in Trinidad." *The Journal of American Folklore* 79 (1966): 537–50.

———. *Black Religions in the New World.* New York: Columbia University Press, 1978.

———. *Religious Cults of the Caribbean: Trinidad, Jamaica, and Haiti.* Rio Piedras: University of Puerto Rico, Institute of Caribbean Studies, 1970.

———. *The Shango Cult in Trinidad.* Rio Piedras: University of Puerto Rico, Institute of Caribbean Studies, 1965.

Sims, Patsy. *Can Somebody Shout Amen! Inside the Tents and Tabernacles of American Revivalists.* Lexington: University of Kentucky Press, 1996.

Smith, Marian W. "The Puyallup-Nisqually." *Columbia University Contributions to Anthropology* 43 (1940).

——. "Shamanism in the Shakers Religion of North America." *Man: The Journal of the Royal Anthropological Institute* 54 (1954): 119–22.

Snyder, Gary. *The Practice of the Wild*. New York: North Point Press, 1990.

——. *Turtle Island*. New York: New Directions, 1974.

Sobel, Mechal. *Trabelin' On*. Princeton, N.J.: Princeton University Press, 1988.

Southey, Robert. *Life of Wesley*. Oxford: Oxford University Press, 1925.

Sovatsky, Stuart. *Eros, Consciousness, and Kundalini: Deepening Sensuality through Tantric Celibacy and Spiritual Intimacy*. Rochester, Vt.: Inner Traditions, 1994.

——. *Words from the Soul: Time, East/West Spirituality, and Psychotherapeutic Narrative*. Albany: State University of New York Press, 1998.

Spencer, Jon Michael. *Protest and Praise: Sacred Music of Black Religion*. Minneapolis: Fortress Press, 1990.

St. Romain, Philip. *Kundalini Energy and Christian Spirituality*. New York: Crossroad, 1995.

Stephens, Patricia. *The Spiritual Baptist Faith: African New World Religious Identity, History and Testimony*. London: Karnak, 1999.

Stuernagel. "Being Filled with the Spirit: The Melodies of Heaven Overflow in the Soul." *The Latter Rain Evangel* 20, no. 10 (1928): 8.

Swedenborg, Emmanuel. *Swedenborg's Journal of Dreams, 1743–1744*. Edited by G. E. Klemmon. New York: Swedenborg Foundation, 1977.

Sweet, William. *Religion of the American Frontier: The Baptists, 1783–1830*. New York, 1931.

Taussig, Michael. *Shamanism, Colonialism, and the Wild Man: A Study in Terror and Healing*. Chicago: The University of Chicago Press, 1987.

Taylor, Rogan. *The Death and Resurrection Show: From Shaman to Superstar*. London: Anthon Bond, 1985.

Testimonies of the Life, Character, Revelations and Doctrines of Mother Ann Lee, and the Elders with Her. Albany: Weed, Parsons & Co., 1888.

Thomas, Nigel H. *Spirits in the Dark*. Concord, Ontario: House of Anansi Press, 1993.

Thompson, Darryl. "The Shakers and Indian Shakers." *The Shaker Messenger* 17 (1995): 5–22.

Thorpe, Margaret Newbold. "Life in Virginia (by a Yankee Teacher)." College of William and Mary: Special Collections Division, Williamsburg, Virginia, 1907.

Torgovnick, Marianna. *Primitive Passions: Men, Women, and the Quest for Ecstasy*. Chicago: The University of Chicago Press, 1996.

Torrance, Robert M. *The Spiritual Quest: Transcendence in Myth, Religion, and Science*. Berkeley: University of California Press, 1994.

Valory, Dale. "The Focus of Indian Shaker Healing." *The Kroeber Anthropological Society Papers* (1966): 69–112.

Van Dusen, Wilson. *The Presence of Other Worlds*. New York: Chrysalis Books, 1974.

Varela, Francisco J. *Ethical Know-How: Action, Wisdom, and Cognition.* Stanford, Calif.: Stanford University Press, 1999.

———. "Not One, Not Two." *CoEvolution Quarterly* 11 (1971): 62–67.

Varela, Francisco J., Evan Thompson, and Eleanor Rosch. *The Embodied Mind: Cognitive Science and Human Experience.* Cambridge, Mass.: The MIT Press, 1999.

Von Foerster, Heinz. *Cybernetics of Cybernetics.* Urbana: University of Illinois, 1974.

———. *Observing Systems.* Seaside, Calif.: Intersystems Publications, 1981.

Wallis, Robert J. *Shamans and Neo-Shamans: Ecstasy, Alternative Archaeologies and Contemporary Pagans.* New York: Routledge, 2003.

Walljasper, Jay. "The Luckiest Man in the World? Bradford Keeney Travels the Globe in Search of the Secrets of Soul." *Utne Magazine* (July–August 2003): 46–54.

Ward, Colleen, and Michael Beaubrun. "Trance Induction and Hallucination in Spiritual Baptists Mourning." *The Journal of Psychological Anthropology* 2 (1979): 479–88.

Waterman, T. T. "The Paraphernalia of the Duwamish 'Spirit-Canoe' Ceremony." *Indian Notes* 7 (1930): 129–48, 535–61.

Waters, Frank. *Book of the Hopi.* Middlesex, England: Penguin, 1963.

Weber, Max. *The Protestant Ethic and the Spirit of Capitalism.* New York: Charles Scribner's Sons, 1930.

Weil, Andrew. *Spontaneous Healing.* New York: Alfred A. Knopf, 1995.

Whitaker, Carl. *From Psyche to System: The Evolving Therapy of Carl Whitaker.* Edited by J. R. Neill and D. P. Kniskern. New York: The Guilford Press, 1982.

———. "Psychotherapy of the Absurd." *Family Process* 14 (1975): 1–16.

Whitaker, Carl, and A. Napier. *The Family Crucible.* New York: Harper and Row, 1978.

White, John, ed. *Kundalini, Evolution and Enlightenment.* New York: Paragon House, 1990.

Whittington, Viola-Gopaul. *History of the Spiritual Baptist and Writings.* Port of Spain, Trinidad: Printing Plus, 1983.

Willett, Henry. "Voices Raised, Singing Praise: Two Centuries of Sacred Sounds in Alamaba." *Alabama Arts* (1995): 13.

Work, John Wesley. *Folk Song of the American Negro.* New York: Negro University Press, 1969.

Yogananda, Paramahansa. *Autobiography of a Yogi.* Los Angeles: Self-Realization Fellowship, 1946.

Yount, David. "Why Did the Quakers Stop Quaking?" *Quaker Life* (March 2002).

Zane, Wallace W. *Journeys to the Spirit Lands: The Natural History of a West Indian Religion.* New York: Oxford University Press, 1999.

INDEX